Alprazolam & Benzodiazepine
A Reference Guide

Contents

1 Alprazolam & Benzodiazepine Overview   **1**
- 1.1 Alprazolam 1
  - 1.1.1 Medical uses 1
  - 1.1.2 Pregnancy and lactation 2
  - 1.1.3 Contraindications 2
  - 1.1.4 Adverse effects 2
  - 1.1.5 Detection in body fluids 5
  - 1.1.6 Pharmacology 5
  - 1.1.7 Pharmacokinetics 5
  - 1.1.8 Forms of alprazolam 5
  - 1.1.9 Synthesis 6
  - 1.1.10 Society and culture 6
  - 1.1.11 References 7
  - 1.1.12 External links 12
- 1.2 Benzodiazepine 12
  - 1.2.1 Medical uses 13
  - 1.2.2 Adverse effects 16
  - 1.2.3 Overdose 18
  - 1.2.4 Contraindications 19
  - 1.2.5 Interactions 20
  - 1.2.6 Pharmacology 20
  - 1.2.7 Pharmacokinetics 22
  - 1.2.8 History 22
  - 1.2.9 Recreational use 23
  - 1.2.10 Veterinary use 24
  - 1.2.11 References 24
  - 1.2.12 External links 31
- 1.3 Anxiolytic 31
  - 1.3.1 Alternatives to medication 31

		1.3.2	Medications	32
		1.3.3	See also	34
		1.3.4	References	35

2 Related Articles & Precautions — 37

2.1 Benzodiazepine overdose — 37
- 2.1.1 Signs and symptoms — 37
- 2.1.2 Toxicity — 38
- 2.1.3 Pathophysiology — 38
- 2.1.4 Diagnosis — 38
- 2.1.5 Treatment — 38
- 2.1.6 Epidemiology — 39
- 2.1.7 References — 40

2.2 Benzodiazepine dependence — 42
- 2.2.1 Definition — 43
- 2.2.2 Signs and symptoms — 43
- 2.2.3 Cause — 43
- 2.2.4 Mechanism — 43
- 2.2.5 Prevention — 46
- 2.2.6 Diagnosis — 46
- 2.2.7 In the elderly — 47
- 2.2.8 Treatment and prevention — 47
- 2.2.9 Epidemiology — 49
- 2.2.10 History — 49
- 2.2.11 Misuse and addiction — 50
- 2.2.12 See also — 50
- 2.2.13 References — 50
- 2.2.14 External links — 54

2.3 Benzodiazepine withdrawal syndrome — 55
- 2.3.1 Signs and symptoms — 55
- 2.3.2 Mechanism — 57
- 2.3.3 Diagnosis — 58
- 2.3.4 Prevention — 58
- 2.3.5 Management — 58
- 2.3.6 Prognosis — 60
- 2.3.7 Epidemiology — 61
- 2.3.8 Special populations — 61
- 2.3.9 Controversy — 63
- 2.3.10 See also — 63

		2.3.11	References	63
		2.3.12	External links	70
	2.4	Benzodiazepine misuse		70
		2.4.1	Background	70
		2.4.2	Health related complications	71
		2.4.3	Rates of misuse	71
		2.4.4	Risk factors for misuse	72
		2.4.5	Drug dependence and withdrawal effects	72
		2.4.6	Drug-related crime	73
		2.4.7	Drug regulation and enforcement	73
		2.4.8	Legal status	74
		2.4.9	See also	74
		2.4.10	References	74
	2.5	Effects of long-term benzodiazepine use		77
		2.5.1	Symptoms	77
		2.5.2	History	80
		2.5.3	Special populations	83
		2.5.4	See also	84
		2.5.5	References	84
3	**Text and image sources, contributors, and licenses**			**89**
	3.1	Text		89
	3.2	Images		92
	3.3	Content license		93

Chapter 1

Alprazolam & Benzodiazepine Overview

1.1 Alprazolam

Alprazolam /æl'præzəlæm/ or /æl'preɪzəlæm/, available as the trade name **Xanax** /'zænæks/ among others, is a short-acting anxiolytic of the benzodiazepine class. It is commonly used for the treatment of panic disorder, and anxiety disorders, such as generalized anxiety disorder (GAD) or social anxiety disorder (SAD).[3][4] It was the 12th most prescribed medicine in 2010.[5] Alprazolam, like other benzodiazepines, binds to specific sites on the GABAA receptor. It possesses anxiolytic, sedative, hypnotic, skeletal muscle relaxant, anticonvulsant, and amnestic properties.[6] Alprazolam is available for oral administration in compressed tablet (CT) and extended-release capsule (XR) formulations.

Alprazolam has a fast onset of action and symptomatic relief. Ninety percent of peak effects are achieved within the first hour of using either the CT formulation or the XR formulation in preparation for panic disorder, and full peak effects are achieved in 1.5 and 1.6 hours respectively.[7][8] Peak benefits achieved for generalized anxiety disorder (GAD) may take up to a week.[9][10] Tolerance to the anxiolytic/antipanic effects is controversial with some authoritative sources reporting the development of tolerance,[11] and others reporting no development of tolerance;[3][12] tolerance will, however, develop to the sedative-hypnotic effects within a couple of days.[12] Withdrawal symptoms or rebound symptoms may occur after ceasing treatment abruptly following a few weeks or longer of steady dosing, and may necessitate a gradual dose reduction.[9][13]

Alprazolam was first released by Upjohn (now a part of Pfizer). It is covered under U.S. Patent 3,987,052, which was filed on 29 October 1969, granted on 19 October 1976, and expired in September 1993. Alprazolam was released in 1981.[14] The first approved indication was panic disorder and within two years of its original marketing Upjohn's Xanax became a blockbuster drug in the US. Presently, Alprazolam is the most prescribed[15] and the most misused benzodiazepine on the U.S. retail market.[16] The potential for misuse among those taking it for medical reasons is controversial with some expert reviews stating that the risk is low and similar to that of other benzodiazepine drugs[3] and others stating that there is a substantial risk of misuse and dependence in both patients and non-medical users of alprazolam and that the pharmacological properties of alprazolam, high affinity binding, high potency, having a short elimination half-life as well as a rapid onset of action may increase the misuse potential of alprazolam.[11][17] Compared to the large number of prescriptions, relatively few individuals increase their dose on their own initiative or engage in drug-seeking behavior.[18] Alprazolam is classified as a schedule IV controlled substance by the U.S. Drug Enforcement Administration (DEA).

1.1.1 Medical uses

Alprazolam is mostly used to treat anxiety disorders, panic disorders, and nausea due to chemotherapy.[17] The FDA label advises that the physician should periodically reassess the usefulness of the drug.[4] Alprazolam may also be indicated for the treatment of generalized anxiety disorder, as well as for the treatment of anxiety conditions with co-morbid depression.[19] Alprazolam is also often prescribed with instances of hypersomnia and co-morbid sleep deficits.

Panic disorder

Alprazolam is effective in the relief of moderate to severe anxiety and panic attacks.[4] However, it is not a first line treatment since the development of selective serotonin reuptake inhibitors, and alprazolam is no longer recommended in Australia for the treatment of panic disorder due to concerns regarding tolerance, dependence and abuse.[11] Evidence supporting the effectiveness of alprazolam in treating panic disorder has been limited to 4 to 10 weeks. However, people with panic disorder have been treated on an open basis for up to 8 months without apparent loss of benefit.[4][20]

In the United States, alprazolam is FDA-approved for the treatment of panic disorder with or without agoraphobia.[4] Alprazolam is recommended by the World Federation of Societies of Biological Psychiatry (WFSBP) for treatment-resistant cases of panic disorder where there is no history of tolerance or dependence.[21]

Anxiety disorders

Anxiety associated with depression is responsive to alprazolam. Demonstrations of the effectiveness by systematic clinical study are limited to 4 months duration for anxiety disorder.[4] However, the research into antidepressant properties of alprazolam is of poor quality and only assessed the short-term effects of alprazolam against depression.[22] In one study, some long term, high-dosage users of alprazolam developed reversible depression.[23] In the US, alprazolam is FDA-approved for the management of anxiety disorders (a condition corresponding most closely to the APA *Diagnostic and Statistical Manual* DSM-IV-TR diagnosis of generalized anxiety disorder) or the short-term relief of symptoms of anxiety. In the UK, alprazolam is recommended for the short-term treatment (2–4 weeks) of severe acute anxiety.[20][24][25]

Nausea due to chemotherapy

Alprazolam may be used in combination with other medications for chemotherapy-induced nausea and vomiting.[17]

1.1.2 Pregnancy and lactation

Benzodiazepines cross the placenta, enter into the fetus and are also excreted with breast milk. The use of benzodiazepines during pregnancy or lactation has potential risks. The use of alprazolam in pregnancy is believed to be associated with congenital abnormalities.

Women who are pregnant or are planning on becoming pregnant should avoid starting alprazolam.[26] Use in the last trimester may cause fetal drug dependence and withdrawal symptoms in the post-natal period[27] as well as neonatal flaccidity and respiratory problems.[28] However, in long-term users of benzodiazepines abrupt discontinuation due to concerns of teratogenesis has a high risk of causing extreme withdrawal symptoms and a severe rebound effect of the underlying mental health disorder. Spontaneous abortions may also result from abrupt withdrawal of psychotropic medications including benzodiazepines.[29]

Benzodiazepines, including alprazolam, are known to be excreted in human milk.[30] Chronic administration of diazepam, another benzodiazepine, to nursing mothers has been reported to cause their infants to become lethargic and to lose weight.[31][32]

1.1.3 Contraindications

Benzodiazepines require special precaution if used in children and in alcohol- or drug-dependent individuals. Particular care should be taken in pregnant or elderly patients, patients with substance abuse history, particularly alcohol dependence and patients with comorbid psychiatric disorders.[33] Use of alprazolam should be avoided or carefully monitored by medical professionals in individuals with the following conditions: myasthenia gravis, acute narrow-angle glaucoma, severe liver deficiencies (e.g., cirrhosis), severe sleep apnea, pre-existing respiratory depression, marked neuromuscular respiratory weakness including unstable myasthenia gravis, acute pulmonary insufficiency, chronic psychosis, hypersensitivity or allergy to alprazolam or other drugs in the benzodiazepine class, borderline personality disorder (may induce suicidality and dyscontrol).[25][34][35]

Like all central nervous system depressants, including alcohol, alprazolam in larger-than-normal doses can cause significant deterioration in alertness, combined with increased feelings of drowsiness, especially in those unaccustomed to the drug's effects.[36] People driving or conducting activities that require vigilance should exercise caution in using alprazolam or any other depressant until they know how it affects them.

Elderly individuals should be cautious in the use of alprazolam due to the possibility of increased susceptibility to side-effects, especially loss of coordination and drowsiness.[31]

1.1.4 Adverse effects

Allergic reactions are unlikely to occur. The only common side effect is sleepiness when treatment is initiated.

Possible side effects include:

- Disinhibition[37]
- Jaundice (very rare)[38]
- Hallucinations (rare)[39]
- Dry mouth (infrequent)[40]
- Ataxia, slurred speech[41]
- Suicidal ideation (rare)[34][42]
- Urinary retention (infrequent)[43]

1.1. ALPRAZOLAM

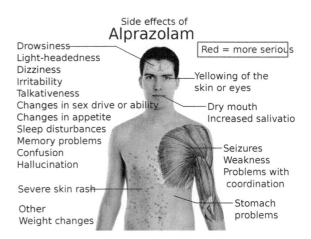

Side effects from Alprazolam

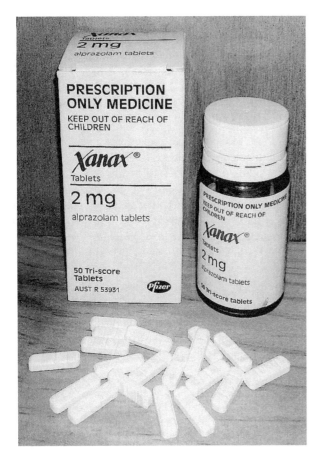

Xanax (alprazolam) 2 mg tri-score tablets

- Skin rash, respiratory depression, constipation[44][45]
- Anterograde amnesia[46] and concentration problems
- Drowsiness, dizziness, lightheadedness, fatigue, unsteadiness and impaired coordination, vertigo[44][45]

Paradoxical reactions

Although unusual, the following paradoxical reactions have been shown to occur:

- Aggression[47]
- Rage, hostility[37]
- Twitches and tremor[48]
- Mania, agitation, hyperactivity and restlessness[49][50][51]

Food and drug interactions

Alprazolam is primarily metabolised via CYP3A4.[52] Combining CYP3A4 inhibitors such as cimetidine, erythromycin, norfluoxetine, fluvoxamine, itraconazole, ketoconazole, nefazodone, propoxyphene, and ritonavir delay the hepatic clearance of alprazolam, which may result in excessive accumulation of alprazolam.[53] This may result in exacerbation of its adverse effect profile.[54][55]

Imipramine and desipramine have been reported to be increased an average of 31% and 20%, respectively, by the concomitant administration of alprazolam tablets in doses up to 4 mg/day.[56] Combined oral contraceptive pills reduce the clearance of alprazolam, which may lead to increased plasma levels of alprazolam and accumulation.[57]

Alcohol is one of the most important and common interactions. Alcohol and benzodiazepines such as alprazolam taken in combination have a synergistic effect on one another, which can cause severe sedation, behavioral changes, and intoxication. The more alcohol and alprazolam taken the worse the interaction.[37] Combination of alprazolam with the herb kava can result in the development of a semi-comatose state.[58] Hypericum conversely can lower the plasma levels of alprazolam and reduce its therapeutic effect.[59][60][61]

Overdose

Main article: Benzodiazepine overdose

Overdoses of alprazolam can be mild to severe depending on how much of the drug is taken and any other drugs that have been taken.[62]

Alprazolam overdoses cause excess central nervous system (CNS) depression and may include one or more of the following symptoms:[43]

- Somnolence (drowsiness)

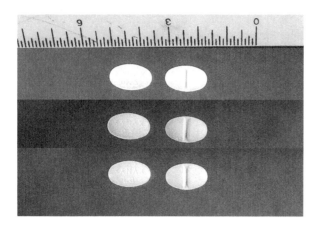

Xanax 0.25, 0.5 and 1 mg scored tablets

- Hypotension (low blood pressure)
- Orthostatic hypotension (fainting while standing up too quickly)
- Hypoventilation (shallow breathing)
- Impaired motor functions
  - Dizziness
  - Impaired balance
  - Muscle weakness
  - Impaired or absent reflexes
- Fainting
- Coma and death are possible if alprazolam is combined with other substances.

Dependence and withdrawal

See also: Benzodiazepine dependence and Benzodiazepine withdrawal syndrome

Alprazolam, like other benzodiazepines, binds to specific sites on the GABAA gamma-amino-butyric acid receptor. When bound to these sites, which are referred to as benzodiazepine receptors, it modulates the effect of GABA A receptors and, thus, GABAergic neurons. Long-term use causes adaptive changes in the benzodiazepine receptors, making them less sensitive to stimulation and less powerful in their effects.[63]

Withdrawal and rebound symptoms commonly occur and necessitate a gradual reduction in dosage to minimize withdrawal effects when discontinuing.[9]

Not all withdrawal effects are evidence of true dependence or withdrawal. Recurrence of symptoms such as anxiety may simply indicate that the drug was having its expected anti-anxiety effect and that, in the absence of the drug, the symptom has returned to pretreatment levels. If the symptoms are more severe or frequent, the patient may be experiencing a rebound effect due to the removal of the drug. Either of these can occur without the patient's actually being drug-dependent.[63]

Alprazolam and other benzodiazepines may also cause the development of physical dependence, tolerance, and benzodiazepine withdrawal symptoms during rapid dose reduction or cessation of therapy after long-term treatment.[64][65] There is a higher chance of withdrawal reactions if the drug is administered in a higher dosage than recommended, or if a patient stops taking the medication altogether without slowly allowing the body to adjust to a lower-dosage regimen.[66][67]

In 1992, Romach and colleagues reported that dose escalation is not a characteristic of long-term alprazolam users, and that the majority of long-term alprazolam users change their initial pattern of regular use to one of symptom control only when required.[68]

Some common symptoms of alprazolam discontinuation include malaise, weakness, insomnia, tachycardia, lightheadedness, and dizziness.[69]

Patients taking a dosing regimen larger than 4 mg per day have an increased potential for dependence. This medication may cause withdrawal symptoms upon abrupt withdrawal or rapid tapering, which in some cases have been known to cause seizures. The discontinuation of this medication may also cause a reaction called *rebound anxiety*.

Delirium similar to that produced by the tropane alkaloids (gaba antagonists) of Datura (scolopamine and atropine) and seizures have been reported in the medical literature from abrupt alprazolam discontinuation.[70][71][72]

In a 1983 study of patients who had taken long-acting benzodiazepines, e.g., clorazepate, for extended periods, the medications were stopped abruptly. Only 5% of patients who had been taking the drug for less than 8 months demonstrated withdrawal symptoms, but 43% of those who had been taking them for more than 8 months did. With alprazolam – a short-acting benzodiazepine – taken for 8 weeks, 65% of patients experienced significant rebound anxiety. To some degree, these older benzodiazepines are self-tapering.[73]

The benzodiazepines diazepam (Valium) and oxazepam (Serepax) have been found to produce fewer withdrawal reactions than alprazolam (Xanax), temazepam (Restoril/Normison), or lorazepam (Temesta/Ativan). Factors that determine the risk of psychological dependence or physical dependence and the severity of the benzodiazepine withdrawal symptoms experienced during dose reduction of alprazolam include: dosage used, length of use, frequency of dosing, personality characteristics of the individual, previous use of cross-dependent/cross-tolerant drugs (alcohol or other sedative-hypnotic drugs), current use of cross-dependent/-tolerant drugs, use of other short-acting, high-potency benzodiazepines,[74][75] and method of discontinuation.[66]

1.1.5 Detection in body fluids

Alprazolam may be quantitated in blood or plasma to confirm a diagnosis of poisoning in hospitalized patients, provide evidence in an impaired driving arrest or to assist in a medicolegal death investigation. Blood or plasma alprazolam concentrations are usually in a range of 10–100 µg/L in persons receiving the drug therapeutically, 100–300 µg/L in those arrested for impaired driving and 300–2000 µg/L in victims of acute overdosage. Most commercial immunoassays for the benzodiazepine class of drugs will cross-react with alprazolam, but confirmation and quantitation is usually performed using chromatographic techniques.[76][77][78]

1.1.6 Pharmacology

Alprazolam is classed as a high-potency benzodiazepine and is a triazolobenzodiazepine,[79][80] namely a benzodiazepine with a triazole ring attached to its structure. Benzodiazepines produce a variety of therapeutic and adverse effects by binding to the benzodiazepine receptor site on the GABAA receptor and modulating the function of the GABA receptor, the most prolific inhibitory receptor within the brain. The GABA chemical and receptor system mediates inhibitory or calming effects of alprazolam on the nervous system. The GABAA receptor is made up of 5 subunits out of a possible 19, and GABAA receptors made up of different combinations of subunits, have different properties, different locations within the brain, and, importantly, different activities with regard to benzodiazepines.[46][81] Benzodiazepines and in particular alprazolam causes a marked suppression of the hypothalamicpituitary-adrenal axis. The therapeutic properties of alprazolam are similar to other benzodiazepines and include anxiolytic, anticonvulsant, muscle relaxant, hypnotic[82] and amnesic.[6]

Administration of alprazolam, but not lorazepam, has been demonstrated to elicit a statistically significant increase in extracellular dopamine D1 and D2 concentrations in the striatum.[83][84]

1.1.7 Pharmacokinetics

Absorption

Following oral administration, alprazolam is readily absorbed. Peak concentrations in the plasma occur in one to two hours following administration. Plasma levels are proportionate to the dose given; over the dose range of 0.5 to 3.0 mg, peak levels of 8.0 to 37 ng/mL were observed. Using a specific assay methodology, the mean plasma elimination half-life of alprazolam has been found to be about 11.2 hours (range: 6.3 to 26.9 hours) in healthy adults.

Distribution

In vitro, alprazolam is bound (80 percent) to human serum protein. Serum albumin accounts for the majority of the binding.

Metabolism/Elimination

Alprazolam is extensively metabolized in humans, primarily by cytochrome P450 3A4 (Cyp3A4), to two major metabolites in plasma: 4-hydroxyalprazolam and α-hydroxyalprazolam. A benzophenone derived from alprazolam is also found in humans. Half-lives are similar to that of alprazolam. The plasma concentrations of 4-hydroxyalprazolam and α-hydroxyalprazolam relative to unchanged alprazolam concentration were always less than 4%. The reported relative potencies in benzodiazepines receptor binding experiments and in animals models of induced seizure inhibition are 0.2 and 0.66, respectively, for 4-hydroxyalprazolam and α-hydroxyalprazolam. Such low concentrations and lesser potencies of 4-hydroxyalprazolam and α-hydroxyalprazolam suggest that they are unlikely to contribute much to the pharmacological effects of alprazolam. The benzophenone metabolite is essentially inactive.

Alprazolam and its metabolites are excreted primarily in the urine.

1.1.8 Forms of alprazolam

Alprazolam regular release and orally disintegrating tablets are available as 0.25 mg, 0.5 mg, 1 mg, 2 mg strength tablets.[85]

Alprazolam extended release tablets are available as 0.5 mg, 1 mg, 2 mg, and 3 mg strength tablets.

Alprazolam oral solutions are available as 0.5 mg/5 mL and as 1 mg/1 mL oral solutions.

- Active ingredient: alprazolam

- Inactive ingredients: microcrystalline cellulose, corn starch, docusate sodium, povidone, sodium starch glycollate, lactose monohydrate, magnesium stearate, colloidal silicon dioxide and sodium benzoate. In addition, the 0.25 mg tablet contains D&C Yellow No. 10 and the 0.5 mg tablet contains FD&C Yellow No. 6 and D&C Yellow No. 10

1.1.9 Synthesis

Alprazolam is a chemical analog of triazolam that differs by the absence of a chlorine atom in the *o*-position of the 6-phenyl ring. The same scheme that was used to make triazolam can be used to make alprazolam, with the exception that it begins with 2-amino-5-chlorobenzophenone.[86][87][88]

Alprazolam synthesis:[89][90][91] *(cf. Estazolam)*

Another way of making alprazolam has been suggested, which comes from 2,6-dichloro-4-phenylquinoline, the reaction of which with hydrazine gives 6-chloro-2-hydrazino-4-phenylquinoline. Boiling this with triethyl orthoacetate in xylene leads to the heterocyclization into a triazole derivative. The resulting product undergoes oxidative cleavage using sodium periodate and ruthenium dioxide in an acetone–water system to give 2-[4-(3′-methyl-1,2,4-triazolo)]−5-chlorobenzophenone.[92][93][94] Oxymethylation of the last using formaldehyde and subsequent substitution of the resulting hydroxyl group by phosphorus tribromide,gives 2-[4-(3′-methyl-5′-bromomethyl-1,2,4-triazolo)]−5-chlorobenzophenone. Substitution of the bromine atom with an amino group using ammonia and the spontaneous, intramolecular heterocyclization following that reaction gives alprazolam.

1.1.10 Society and culture

Recreational use

See also: Benzodiazepine misuse

There is a risk of misuse and dependence in both patients and non-medical users of alprazolam; the pharmacological properties of alprazolam such as high affinity binding, high potency, being short-acting and having a rapid onset of action increase the abuse potential of alprazolam. The physical dependence and withdrawal syndrome of alprazolam also adds to the addictive nature of alprazolam. In the small subgroup of individuals who escalate their doses there is usually a history of alcohol or other substance use disorders.[11] Despite this, most prescribed alprazolam users do not use their medication recreationally, and the long-term use of benzodiazepines does not generally correlate with the need for dose escalation.[95] However, based on US findings from the Treatment Episode Data Set (TEDS), an annual compilation of patient characteristics in substance abuse treatment facilities in the United States, admissions due to "primary tranquilizer" (including, but not limited to, benzodiazepine-type) drug use increased 79% from 1992 to 2002, suggesting that misuse of benzodiazepines may be on the rise.[96] *The New York Times* also reported in 2011 that "The Centers for Disease Control and Prevention last year reported an 89 percent increase in emergency room visits nationwide related to nonmedical benzodiazepine use between 2004 and 2008."[97]

Alprazolam is one of the most commonly prescribed and misused benzodiazepines in the United States.[13][16] A large-scale nationwide U.S. government study conducted by SAMHSA found that, in the U.S., benzodiazepines are recreationally the most frequently used pharmaceuticals due to their widespread availability, accounting for 35% of all drug-related visits to hospital emergency and urgent care facilities. Men and women are equally likely to use benzodiazepines recreationally. The report found that alprazolam is the most common benzodiazepine for recreational use followed by clonazepam, lorazepam, and diazepam. The number of emergency room visits due to benzodiazepines increased by 36% between 2004 and 2006.[16]

> Regarding the significant increases detected, it is worthwhile to consider that the number of pharmaceuticals dispensed for legitimate therapeutic uses may be increasing over time, and DAWN estimates are not adjusted to take such increases into account. Nor do DAWN estimates take into account the increases in the population or in ED use between 2004 and 2006.[16]

At a particularly high risk for misuse and dependence are people with a history of alcoholism or drug abuse and/or dependence[98][99] and people with borderline personality disorder.[100]

Alprazolam, along with other benzodiazepines, is often used with other recreational drugs. These uses include aids to relieve the panic or distress of dysphoric ("bad trip") reactions to psychedelic drugs, such as LSD, and the drug-induced agitation and insomnia in the "comedown" stages of stimulant use, such as amphetamine, cocaine, and phencyclidine allowing sleep. Alprazolam may also be used in conjunction with other depressant drugs, such as ethanol, heroin and other opioids, in an attempt to enhance the psychological effect of these drugs. Alprazolam may be used in conjunction with cannabis, with users citing a synergistic effect achieved after consuming the combination.

The poly-drug use of powerful depressant drugs poses the highest level of health concerns due to a significant increase in the likelihood of experiencing an overdose which may result in fatal respiratory depression.[101][102]

A 1990 study claimed that diazepam has a higher misuse potential relative to other benzodiazepines, and that some data suggests that alprazolam and lorazepam resemble diazepam in this respect.[103]

Anecdotally injection of alprazolam has been reported, causing dangerous damage to blood vessels, closure of blood vessels (embolization) and decay of muscle tissue (rhabdomyolysis).[104] Alprazolam is practically not soluble in water, when crushed in water it will not fully dissolve (40 μg/ml of H_2O at pH 7).[105] There have also been anecdotal reports of alprazolam being snorted.[106] Due to the low weight of a dose, alprazolam in one case was found to be distributed on blotter paper in a manner similar to LSD.[107]

Slang terms for alprazolam vary from place to place. Some of the more common terms are shortened versions of the trade name "Xanax", such as Bars or Zannies; references to their drug classes, such as benzos or downers; or remark upon their shape or color (most commonly a straight, perforated tablet or an oval-shaped pill): bars, Z-bars, footballs, planks, blues, or blue footballs.[108][109][110]

Availability

Alprazolam is available in English-speaking countries under the following brand names:[111]

- Alprax, Alprocontin, Alzam, Alzolam, Anzilum, Apo-Alpraz, Kalma, Mylan-Alprazolam, Niravam, Novo-Alprazol, Nu-Alpraz, Pacyl, Restyl, Tranax, Trika, Xycalm, Xanax, Xanor, Zolam, Zopax, Helex.

As of December 2013, in anticipation of the rescheduling of alprazolam to Schedule 8 in Australia—Pfizer Australia announced they would be discontinuing the Xanax brand in Australia as it is no longer commercially viable.[112]

Legal status

In the United States, alprazolam is a prescription drug and is assigned to Schedule IV of the Controlled Substances Act by the Drug Enforcement Administration.[113] Under the UK drug misuse classification system benzodiazepines are class C drugs (Schedule 4).[114] In the UK, alprazolam is not available on the NHS and can only be obtained on a private prescription.[115] Internationally, alprazolam is included under the United Nations Convention on Psychotropic Substances as Schedule IV.[116] In Ireland, alprazolam is a Schedule 4 medicine.[117] In Sweden, alprazolam is a prescription drug in List IV (Schedule 4) under the Narcotics Drugs Act (1968).[118] In the Netherlands, alprazolam is a List 2 substance of the Opium Law and is available for prescription. In Australia, alprazolam was originally a Schedule 4 (Prescription Only) medication; however, as of February 2014, it has become a Schedule 8 medication, subjecting it to more rigorous prescribing requirements.[119]

1.1.11 References

[1] "Xanax (Alprazolam) Clinical Pharmacology – Prescription Drugs and Medications". *RxList*. First DataBank. July 2008.

[2] "Xanax XR (Alprazolam) Clinical Pharmacology – Prescription Drugs and Medications". *RxList*. First DataBank. July 2008.

[3] Work Group on Panic Disorder (January 2009). *APA Practice Guideline for the Treatment of Patients With Panic Disorder* (2nd ed.). doi:10.1176/appi.books.9780890423905.154688.

[4] "FDA approved labeling for Xanax revision 08/23/2011" (PDF). Federal Drug Administration. 2011-08-23. p. 4. Retrieved 2011-09-14. Anxiety Disorders – XANAX Tablets (alprazolam) are indicated for the management of anxiety disorder (a condition corresponding most closely to the APA Diagnostic and Statistical Manual [DSMIII-R] diagnosis of generalized anxiety disorder) or the short-term relief of symptoms of anxiety. Anxiety or tension associated with the stress of everyday life usually does not require treatment with an anxiolytic... Panic Disorder – XANAX is also indicated for the treatment of panic disorder, with or without agoraphobia... Demonstrations of the effectiveness of XANAX by systematic clinical study are limited to 4 months duration for anxiety disorder and 4 to 10 weeks duration for panic disorder; however, patients with panic disorder have been treated on an open basis without any apparent loss of benefit. The physician should periodically reassess the usefulness of the drug for the individual patient.

[5] "In Pictures: The Most Popular Prescription Drugs". *Forbes*. Retrieved 2015-06-16.

[6] Mandrioli, R.; Mercolini, L.; Raggi, M. A. (2008). "Benzodiazepine Metabolism: An Analytical Perspective". *Current Drug Metabolism* **9** (8): 827–844. doi:10.2174/138920008786049258. PMID 18855614.

[7] Sheehan, D. V.; Sheehan, K. H.; Raj, B. A. (2007). "The Speed of Onset of Action of Alprazolam-XR Compared to Alprazolam-CT in Panic Disorder". *Psychopharmacology Bulletin* **40** (2): 63–81. PMID 17514187.

[8] Smith, R. B.; Kroboth, P. D.; Vanderlugt, J. T.; Phillips, J. P.; Juhl, R. P. (1984). "Pharmacokinetics and Pharmacodynamics of Alprazolam after Oral and IV Administration". *Psychopharmacology* **84** (4): 452–456. doi:10.1007/bf00431449. PMID 6152055.

[9] Verster, J. C.; Volkerts, E. R. (2004). "Clinical Pharmacology, Clinical Efficacy, and Behavioral Toxicity of Alprazolam: A Review of the Literature" (PDF). *CNS Drug Reviews* **10** (1): 45–76. doi:10.1111/j.1527-3458.2004.tb00003.x. PMID 14978513.

[10] Tampi, R. R.; Muralee, S.; Weder, N. D.; Penland, H., eds. (2008). *Comprehensive Review of Psychiatry*. Philadelphia, PA: Wolters Kluwer / Lippincott Williams & Wilkins Health. p. 226. ISBN 978-0-7817-7176-4. Retrieved 2014-01-22.

[11] Moylan, S.; Giorlando, F.; Nordfjærn, T.; Berk, M. (2012). "The Role of Alprazolam for the Treatment of Panic Disorder in Australia" (PDF). *The Australian and New Zealand Journal of Psychiatry* **46** (3): 212–224. doi:10.1177/0004867411432074. PMID 22391278.

[12] Pavuluri, M. N.; Janicak, P. G.; Marder, S. R. (2010). *Principles and Practice of Psychopharmacotherapy* (5th ed.). Philadelphia, PA: Wolters Kluwer Health / Lippincott Williams & Wilkins. p. 535. ISBN 978-1-60547-565-3. Retrieved 2014-01-22.

[13] Galanter, M. (2008). *The American Psychiatric Publishing Textbook of Substance Abuse Treatment* (4th ed.). American Psychiatric Publishing. p. 222. ISBN 978-1-58562-276-4. Retrieved 2014-01-22.

[14] Walker, S. (1996). *A Dose of Sanity: Mind, Medicine, and Misdiagnosis*. New York: John Wiley & Sons. pp. 64–65. ISBN 978-0-471-19262-6.

[15] Langreth, Robert; Herper, Matthew (2010-05-11). "In Pictures: The Most Popular Prescription Drugs". Forbes.

[16] "Drug Abuse Warning Network, 2006: National Estimates of Drug-Related Emergency Department Visits" (PDF). *U.S. Department of Health and Human Services*. Substance Abuse and Mental Health Services Administration. 2006. Retrieved 13 February 2012.

[17] "Alprazolam". *The American Society of Health-System Pharmacists*. Archived from the original on 15 May 2011. Retrieved 3 April 2011.

[18] "DEA Brief Benzodiazepines". Archived from the original on 2009-03-12. Retrieved 1 October 2011. Given the millions of prescriptions written for benzodiazepines (about 100 million in 1999), relatively few individuals increase their dose on their own initiative or engage in drug-seeking behavior.

[19] "Xanax (Alprazolam) Drug Information: Indications, Dosage and How Supplied – Prescribing Information". *Rxlist.com*. RxList. Retrieved 2013-09-20.

[20] "Xanax (Alprazolam) Clinical Pharmacology – Prescription Drugs and Medications at RxList". *RxList*. First DataBank. July 2008.

[21] Bandelow, B.; Zohar, J.; Hollander, E.; Kasper, S.; Möller, H. J.; WFSBP Task Force On Treatment Guidelines For Anxiety, O. C. P. S. D. (2002). "World Federation of Societies of Biological Psychiatry (WFSBP) Guidelines for the Pharmacological Treatment of Anxiety, Obsessive-Compulsive and Posttraumatic Stress Disorders". *World Journal of Biological Psychiatry* **3** (4): 171–199. doi:10.3109/15622970209150621. PMID 12516310.

[22] van Marwijk, H.; Allick, G.; Wegman, F.; Bax, A.; Riphagen, I. I. (2012). van Marwijk, Harm, ed. "Alprazolam for depression". *Cochrane Database Syst Rev* **7**: CD007139. doi:10.1002/14651858.CD007139.pub2. PMID 22786504.

[23] Lydiard, R. B.; Laraia, M. T.; Ballenger, J. C.; Howell, E. F. (May 1987). "Emergence of Depressive Symptoms in Patients Receiving Alprazolam for Panic Disorder". *The American Journal of Psychiatry* **144** (5): 664–665. doi:10.1176/ajp.144.5.664. PMID 3578580.

[24] "Xanax". *Netdoctor.co.uk*. NetDoctor. 2006-10-01. Archived from the original on 9 August 2007. Retrieved 2007-08-02.

[25] "Alprazolam". British National Formulary. 2007. Retrieved 3 August 2007.

[26] "Xanax (Alprazolam) Drug Information: Uses, Side Effects, Drug Interactions and Warnings". *RxList.com*. United States: RxList. July 2008. p. 4.

[27] Iqbal, M. M.; Sobhan, T.; Ryals, T. (2002). "Effects of Commonly Used Benzodiazepines on the Fetus, the Neonate, and the Nursing Infant". *Psychiatric Services* **53** (1): 39–49. doi:10.1176/appi.ps.53.1.39. PMID 11773648.

[28] García-Algar, Ó.; López-Vílchez, M. Á.; Martín, I.; Mur, A.; Pellegrini, M.; Pacifici, R.; Rossi, S.; Pichini, S. (2007). "Confirmation of Gestational Exposure to Alprazolam by Analysis of Biological Matrices in a Newborn with Neonatal Sepsis". *Clinical Toxicology* **45** (3): 295–298. doi:10.1080/15563650601072191. PMID 17453885.

[29] Einarson, A.; Selby, P.; Koren, G. (2001). "Abrupt Discontinuation of Psychotropic Drugs During Pregnancy: Fear of Teratogenic Risk and Impact of Counselling" (PDF). *Journal of Psychiatry and Neuroscience* **26** (1): 44–48. PMC 1408034. PMID 11212593.

[30] Oo, C. Y.; Kuhn, R. J.; Desai, N.; Wright, C. E.; McNamara, P. J. (1995). "Pharmacokinetics in Lactating Women: Prediction of Alprazolam Transfer into Milk". *British Journal of Clinical Pharmacology* **40** (3): 231–236. doi:10.1111/j.1365-2125.1995.tb05778.x. PMC 1365102. PMID 8527284.

[31] "Alprazolam – Oral (Xanax) Side Effects, Medical Uses, and Drug Interactions". *Medicinenet.com*. MedicineNet. July 2005. Archived from the original on 18 December 2008. Retrieved 2008-12-07.

[32] "Xanax (Alprazolam) Drug Information: Uses, Side Effects, Drug Interactions and Warnings". *RxList.com*. RxList. July 2008. p. 8. Archived from the original on 5 December 2008. Retrieved 2008-12-07.

[33] Authier, N.; Balayssac, D.; Sautereau, M.; Zangarelli, A.; Courty, P.; Somogyi, A. A.; et al. (2009). "Benzodiazepine Dependence: Focus on Withdrawal Syndrome". *Annales Pharmaceutiques Françaises* **67** (6): 408–413. doi:10.1016/j.pharma.2009.07.001. PMID 19900604.

[34] Hori, A. (1998). "Pharmacotherapy for Personality Disorders". *Psychiatry and Clinical Neurosciences* **52** (1): 13–19. doi:10.1111/j.1440-1819.1998.tb00967.x. PMID 9682928.

[35] Gardner, D. L.; Cowdry, R. W. (1985). "Alprazolam-Induced Dyscontrol in Borderline Personality Disorder". *American Journal of Psychiatry* **142** (1): 98–100. doi:10.1176/ajp.142.1.98. PMID 2857071.

[36] Kozená, L.; Frantik, E.; Horváth, M. (1995). "Vigilance Impairment after a Single Dose of Benzodiazepines". *Psychopharmacology* **119** (1): 39–45. doi:10.1007/BF02246052. PMID 7675948.

[37] Michel, L.; Lang, J. P. (2003). "Benzodiazépines et passage à l'acte criminel" [Benzodiazepines and Forensic Aspects]. *Encephale* (in French) **29** (6): 479–485. PMID 15029082. Retrieved 9 April 2013.

[38] Noyes, R.; DuPont, R. L.; Pecknold, J. C.; Rifkin, A.; Rubin, R. T.; Swinson, R. P.; et al. (1988). "Alprazolam in Panic Disorder and Agoraphobia: Results from a Multicenter Trial. II. Patient Acceptance, Side Effects, and Safety". *Archives of General Psychiatry* **45** (5): 423–428. doi:10.1001/archpsyc.1988.01800290037005. PMID 3358644.

[39] "Complete Alprazolam Information". *Drugs.com*. Archived from the original on 5 August 2007. Retrieved 2 August 2007.

[40] Elie, R.; Lamontagne, Y. (1984). "Alprazolam and Diazepam in the Treatment of Generalized Anxiety". *Journal of Clinical Psychopharmacology* **4** (3): 125–129. doi:10.1097/00004714-198406000-00002. PMID 6145726.

[41] Cassano, G. B.; Toni, C.; Petracca, A.; Deltito, J.; Benkert, O.; Curtis, G.; et al. (1994). "Adverse Effects Associated with the Short-term Treatment of Panic Disorder with Imipramine, Alprazolam or Placebo". *European Neuropsychopharmacology* **4** (1): 47–53. doi:10.1016/0924-977X(94)90314-X. PMID 8204996.

[42] Kravitz, H. M.; Fawcett, J.; Newman, A. J. (1993). "Alprazolam and Depression: A Review of Risks and Benefits". *Journal of Clinical Psychiatry* **54** (Supplement): 78–84; discussion 85. PMID 8262892.

[43] "Alprazolam Side Effects, Interactions and Information". *Drugs.com*. Archived from the original on 19 August 2007. Retrieved 2 August 2007.

[44] Rawson, N. S.; Rawson, M. J. (1999). "Acute Adverse Event Signalling Scheme Using the Saskatchewan Administrative Health Care Utilization Datafiles: Results for Two Benzodiazepines". *Canadian Journal of Clinical Pharmacology* **6** (3): 159–166. PMID 10495368.

[45] "Alprazolam – Complete Medical Information Regarding This Treatment of Anxiety Disorders". *Medicinenet.com*. MedicineNet. Retrieved 2 August 2007.

[46] Barbee, J. G. (1993). "Memory, Benzodiazepines, and Anxiety: Integration of Theoretical and Clinical Perspectives". *The Journal of Clinical Psychiatry* **54** (Suppl): 86–97; discussion 98–101. PMID 8262893.

[47] Rapaport, M.; Braff, D. L. (1985). "Alprazolam and Hostility". *American Journal of Psychiatry* **142** (1): 146. PMID 2857070.

[48] Béchir, M.; Schwegler, K.; Chenevard, R.; Binggeli, C.; Caduff, C.; Büchi, S.; et al. (2007). "Anxiolytic Therapy with Alprazolam Increases Muscle Sympathetic Activity in Patients with Panic Disorders". *Autonomic Neuroscience* **134** (1–2): 69–73. doi:10.1016/j.autneu.2007.01.007. PMID 17363337.

[49] Arana, G. W.; Pearlman, C.; Shader, R. I. (1985). "Alprazolam-Induced Mania: Two Clinical Cases". *American Journal of Psychiatry* **142** (3): 368–369. doi:10.1176/ajp.142.3.368. PMID 2857534.

[50] Strahan, A.; Rosenthal, J.; Kaswan, M.; Winston, A. (1985). "Three Case Reports of Acute Paroxysmal Excitement Associated with Alprazolam Treatment". *American Journal of Psychiatry* **142** (7): 859–861. doi:10.1176/ajp.142.7.859. PMID 2861755.

[51] Reddy, J.; Khanna, S.; Anand, U.; Banerjee, A. (1996). "Alprazolam-Induced Hypomania". *Australia and New Zealand Journal of Psychiatry* **30** (4): 550–552. doi:10.3109/00048679609065031. PMID 8887708.

[52] Otani, K. (2003). "Cytochrome P450 3A4 and Benzodiazepines". *Seishin Shinkeigaku Zasshi* (in Japanese) **105** (5): 631–642. PMID 12875231.

[53] Dresser, G. K.; Spence, J. D.; Bailey, D. G. (2000). "Pharmacokinetic-Pharmacodynamic Consequences and Clinical Relevance of Cytochrome P450 3A4 Inhibition". *Clinical Pharmacokinetics* **38** (1): 41–57. doi:10.2165/00003088-200038010-00003. PMID 10668858.

[54] Greenblatt, D. J.; Wright, C. E. (1993). "Clinical Pharmacokinetics of Alprazolam. Therapeutic Implications". *Clinical Pharmacokinetics* **24** (6): 453–471. doi:10.2165/00003088-199324060-00003. PMID 8513649.

[55] Wang, J. S.; Chase, C. L. (2003). "Pharmacokinetics and Drug Interactions of the Sedative Hypnotics" (PDF). *Psychopharmacological Bulletin* **37** (1): 10–29. doi:10.1007/BF01990373. PMID 14561946. Archived from the original (PDF) on 2007-07-09.

[56] "FDA SPL Approved Application Filing for NDC Code 0228-3083 (Alprazolam by Actavis Elizabeth LLC)".

[57] Back, D. J.; Orme, M. L. (1990). "Pharmacokinetic Drug Interactions with Oral Contraceptives". *Clinical Pharmacokinetics* **18** (6): 472–484. doi:10.2165/00003088-199018060-00004. PMID 2191822.

[58] Izzo, A. A.; Ernst, E. (2001). "Interactions between Herbal Medicines and Prescribed Drugs: A Systematic Review". *Drugs* **61** (15): 2163–2175. doi:10.2165/00003495-200161150-00002. PMID 11772128.

[59] Izzo, A. A. (2004). "Drug Interactions with St. John's Wort (*Hypericum perforatum*): A Review of the Clinical Evidence". *International Journal of Clinical Pharmacology and Therapeutics* **42** (3): 139–148. doi:10.5414/CPP42139. PMID 15049433.

[60] Madabushi, R.; Frank, B.; Drewelow, B.; Derendorf, H.; Butterweck, V. (2006). "Hyperforin in St. John's Wort Drug Interactions". *European Journal of Clinical Pharmacology* **62** (3): 225–233. doi:10.1007/s00228-006-0096-0. PMID 16477470.

[61] Izzo, A. A.; Ernst, E. (2009). "Interactions between Herbal Medicines and Prescribed Drugs: An Updated Systematic Review". *Drugs* **69** (13): 1777–1798. doi:10.2165/11317010-000000000-00000. PMID 19719333.

[62] Isbister, G. K.; O'Regan, L.; Sibbritt, D.; Whyte, I. M. (2004). "Alprazolam is Relatively more Toxic than other Benzodiazepines in Overdose". *British Journal of Clinical Pharmacology* **58** (1): 88–95. doi:10.1111/j.1365-2125.2004.02089.x. PMC 1884537. PMID 15206998.

[63] Stahl, S. (1996). *Essential Pharmacology: Neuroscientific Basis and Practical Applications*. Cambridge: Cambridge University Press. ISBN 0-521-42620-0.

[64] Juergens, S. M.; Morse, R. M. (1988). "Alprazolam Dependence in seven Patients". *The American Journal of Psychiatry* **145** (5): 625–627. doi:10.1176/ajp.145.5.625. PMID 3258735.

[65] Klein, E. (2002). "The Role of Extended-Release Benzodiazepines in the Treatment of Anxiety: A Risk-Benefit Evaluation with a Focus on Extended-Release Alprazolam". *The Journal of Clinical Psychiatry* **63** (Suppl 14): 27–33. PMID 12562116.

[66] Ashton, Heather (August 2002). "The Ashton Manual – Benzodiazepines: How They Work and How to Withdraw". Benzo.org.uk. Retrieved 2008-10-31.

[67] Closser, M. H.; Brower, K. J. (1994). "Treatment of Alprazolam Withdrawal with Chlordiazepoxide Substitution and Taper". *Journal of Substance Abuse Treatment* **11** (4): 319–323. doi:10.1016/0740-5472(94)90042-6. PMID 7966502.

[68] Romach, M. K.; Somer, G. R.; Sobell, L. C.; Sobell, M. B.; Kaplan, H. L.; Sellers, E. M. (1992). "Characteristics of Long-Term Alprazolam Users in the Community". *Journal of Clinical Psychopharmacology* **12** (5): 316–321. doi:10.1097/00004714-199210000-00004. PMID 1479048.

[69] Fyer, A. J.; Liebowitz, M. R.; Gorman, J. M.; Campeas, R.; Levin, A.; Davies, S. O.; et al. (1987). "Discontinuation of Alprazolam Treatment in Panic Patients". *American Journal of Psychiatry* **144** (3): 303–308. doi:10.1176/ajp.144.3.303. PMID 3826428. Retrieved 2008-12-10.

[70] Breier, A.; Charney, D. S.; Nelson, J. C. (1984). "Seizures Induced by Abrupt Discontinuation of Alprazolam". *The American Journal of Psychiatry* **141** (12): 1606–1607. PMID 6150649.

[71] Noyes Jr, R.; Perry, P. J.; Crowe, R. R.; Coryell, W. H.; Clancy, J.; Yamada, T.; Gabel, J. (1986). "Seizures following the withdrawal of alprazolam". *The Journal of Nervous and Mental Disease* **174** (1): 50–52. doi:10.1097/00005053-198601000-00009. PMID 2867122.

[72] Levy, A. B. (1984). "Delirium and Seizures due to Abrupt Alprazolam Withdrawal: Case Report". *The Journal of Clinical Psychiatry* **45** (1): 38–39. PMID 6141159.

[73] Schatzberg, A.; DeBattista, C. (2003). *Manual of Clinical Psychopharmacology*. Washington, DC: American Psychiatric Pub. p. 391. ISBN 1-58562-209-5. Retrieved 2014-01-22.

[74] Wolf, B.; Griffiths, R. R. (1991). "Physical Dependence on Benzodiazepines: Differences Within the Class". *Drug and Alcohol Dependence* **29** (2): 153–156. doi:10.1016/0376-8716(91)90044-Y. PMID 1686752.

[75] Higgitt, A.; Fonagy, P.; Lader, M. (1988). "The Natural History of Tolerance to the Benzodiazepines". *Psychological Medicine. Monograph Supplement* **13**: 1–55. doi:10.1017/S0264180100000412. PMID 2908516.

[76] Jones, A. W.; Holmgren, A.; Kugelberg, F. C. (2007). "Concentrations of Scheduled Prescription Drugs in Blood of Impaired Drivers: Considerations for Interpreting the Results". *Therapeutic Drug Monitoring* **29** (2): 248–260. doi:10.1097/FTD.0b013e31803d3c04. PMID 17417081.

[77] Fraser, A. D.; Bryan, W. (1991). "Evaluation of the Abbott ADx and TDx Serum Benzodiazepine Immunoassays for Analysis of Alprazolam". *Journal of Analytic Toxicology* **15** (2): 63–65. doi:10.1093/jat/15.2.63. PMID 1675703.

[78] Baselt, R. (2011). *Disposition of Toxic Drugs and Chemicals in Man* (9th ed.). Seal Beach, CA: Biomedical Publications. pp. 45–48. ISBN 978-0-9626523-8-7.

[79] Skelton, K. H.; Nemeroff, C. B.; Owens, M. J. (2004). "Spontaneous Withdrawal from the Triazolobenzodiazepine Alprazolam Increases Cortical Corticotropin-Releasing Factor mRNA Expression". *Journal of Neuroscience* **24** (42): 9303–9312. doi:10.1523/JNEUROSCI.1737-04.2004. PMID 15496666.

[80] Chouinard, G. (2004). "Issues in the Clinical Use of Benzodiazepines: Potency, Withdrawal, and Rebound". *Journal of Clinical Psychiatry* **65** (Suppl 5): 7–12. PMID 15078112.

[81] White, G.; Gurley, D. A. (1995). "α Subunits Influence Zn Block of γ2 Containing GABAA Receptor Currents". *NeuroReport* **6** (3): 461–464. doi:10.1097/00001756-199502000-00014. PMID 7766843.

[82] Arvat, E.; Giordano, R.; Grottoli, S.; Ghigo, E. (2002). "Benzodiazepines and Anterior Pituitary Function". *Journal of Endocrinological Investigation* **25** (8): 735–747. doi:10.1007/bf03345110. PMID 12240908.

[83] Bentué-Ferrer, D.; Reymann, J. M.; Tribut, O.; Allain, H.; Vasar, E.; Bourin, M. (2001). "Role of dopaminergic and serotonergic systems on behavioral stimulatory effects of low-dose alprazolam and lorazepam". *European neuropsychopharmacology : the journal of the European College of Neuropsychopharmacology* **11** (1): 41–50. doi:10.1016/S0924-977X(00)00137-1. PMID 11226811.

[84] Giardino, L.; Zanni, M.; Pozza, M.; Bettelli, C.; Covelli, V. (1998-03-05). "Dopamine receptors in the striatum of rats exposed to repeated restraint stress and alprazolam treatment". *European Journal of Pharmacology* **344** (2-3): 143–147. ISSN 0014-2999. PMID 9600648.

[85] "Alprazolam Dosage, Uses, Overdose Info and More". RXwiki.com. November 18, 2013. Retrieved 2014-01-22. (🔊 Page will play audio when loaded)

[86] US patent 3987052, Jackson, H.B.

[87] DE 2012190, Jackson, H.B.

[88] Hester, J. B. Jr.; Duchamp, D. J.; Chidester, C. G. (1971). "A Synthetic Approach to New 1,4-Benzodiazepine Derivatives". *Tetrahedron Letters* **12** (20): 1609–1612. doi:10.1016/S0040-4039(01)87414-1.

[89] Meguro, K.; Natsugari, H.; Tawada, H.; Kuwada, Y. (1973). "Heterocycles. IV. Reactions of 2-Amino-3H-1,4-benzodiazepines with Primary Amines and Hydroxylamines". *Chemical & Pharmaceutical Bulletin* **21** (11): 2366. doi:10.1248/cpb.21.2366.

[90] Meguro, K.; Kuwada, Y. (1973). "Heterocycles. V. Syntheses and Structures of 7-Chloro-2-hydrazino-5-phenyl-3H-1,4-benzodiazepines and Some Isomeric 1,4,5-Benzotriazocines". *Chemical & Pharmaceutical Bulletin* **21** (11): 2375. doi:10.1248/cpb.21.2375.

[91] Meguro, K.; Tawada, H.; Miyano, H.; Sato, Y.; Kuwada, Y. (1973). "Heterocycles. VI. Syntheses of 4H-s-Triazolo[4,3-a][1,4]benzodiazepines, Novel Tricyclic Psychosedatives". *Chemical & Pharmaceutical Bulletin* **21** (11): 2382. doi:10.1248/cpb.21.2382.

[92] Walser, A.; Zenchoff, G. (1977). "Quinazolines and 1,4-Benzodiazepines. 81. s-Triazolo[4,3-a][1,4]benzodiazepines by Oxidative Cyclization of Hydrazones". *Journal of Medicinal Chemistry* **20** (12): 1694–1697. doi:10.1021/jm00222a035. PMID 592339.

[93] US patent 3709898, Hester, J.

[94] US patent 3781289, Hester, J.

[95] Soumerai, S. B.; Simoni-Wastila, L.; Singer, C.; Mah, C.; Gao, X.; Salzman, C.; et al. (2003). "Lack of Relationship between Long-Term Use of Benzodiazepines and Escalation to High Dosages". *Psychiatric Services* **54** (7): 1006–1011. doi:10.1176/appi.ps.54.7.1006. PMID 12851438.

[96] Licata, S. C.; Rowlett, J. K. (2008). "Abuse and Dependence Liability of Benzodiazepine-Type Drugs: GABAA Receptor Modulation and Beyond". *Pharmacology Biochemistry and Behavior* **90** (1): 74–89. doi:10.1016/j.pbb.2008.01.001. PMC 2453238. PMID 18295321.

[97] Goodnough, Abby (September 14, 2011). "Abuse of Xanax Leads a Clinic to Halt Supply". *New York Times*.

[98] Ballenger, J. C. (1984). "Psychopharmacology of the Anxiety Disorders". *The Psychiatric Clinics of North America* **7** (4): 757–771. PMID 6151647.

[99] Ciraulo, D. A.; Barnhill, J. G.; Greenblatt, D. J.; Shader, R. I.; Ciraulo, A. M.; Tarmey, M. F.; Molloy, M. A.; Foti, M. E. (1988). "Abuse Liability and Clinical Pharmacokinetics of Alprazolam in Alcoholic Men". *The Journal of Clinical Psychiatry* **49** (9): 333–337. PMID 3417618.

[100] Vorma, H.; Naukkarinen, H. H.; Sarna, S. J.; Kuoppasalmi, K. I. (2005). "Predictors of Benzodiazepine Discontinuation in Subjects Manifesting Complicated Dependence". *Substance Use & Misuse* **40** (4): 499–510. doi:10.1081/JA-200052433. PMID 15830732.

[101] Walker, B. M.; Ettenberg, A. (2003). "The Effects of Alprazolam on Conditioned Place Preferences Produced by Intravenous Heroin". *Pharmacology, Biochemistry, and Behavior* **75** (1): 75–80. doi:10.1016/S0091-3057(03)00043-1. PMID 12759115.

[102] "OSAM-O-GRAM Highlights of Statewide Drug Use Trends" (PDF). Ohio, US: Wright State University and the University of Akron. January 2008. Retrieved 2008-12-10.

[103] Griffiths, R. R.; Wolf, B. (1990). "Relative Abuse Liability of Different Benzodiazepines in Drug Abusers". *Journal of Clinical Psychopharmacology* **10** (4): 237–243. doi:10.1097/00004714-199008000-00002. PMID 1981067.

[104] Wang, E. C.; Chew, F. S. (2006). "MR Findings of Alprazolam Injection into the Femoral Artery with Microembolization and Rhabdomyolysis" (PDF). *Radiology Case Reports* **1** (3). doi:10.2484/rcr.v1i3.33.

[105] "DB00404 (Alprazolam)". Canada: DrugBank. 2008-06-26. Archived from the original on 6 July 2011. Retrieved 2011-07-12.

[106] Sheehan, M. F.; Sheehan, D. V.; Torres, A.; Coppola, A.; Francis, E. (1991). "Snorting benzodiazepines". *The American Journal of Drug and Alcohol Abuse* **17** (4): 457–468. doi:10.3109/00952999109001605. PMID 1684083.

[107] "INTELLIGENCE ALERT – XANAX BLOTTER PAPER IN BARTLESVILLE, OKLAHOMA" (Microgram Bulletin). US DEA. May 2008. Archived from the original on 2008-05-21.

[108] "Street Terms for Xanax". *Axisresidentialtreatment.com*. Retrieved 2014-02-14.

[109] "Street Names for Alprazolam". *Alprazolamaddictionhelp.com*. Retrieved 2014-02-14.

[110] "Xanax Effects and Withdrawal Symptoms". *Drugrehabtreatmenthelp.com*. 2010. Retrieved 2014-02-14.

[111] "Benzodiazepine Names". Non-benzodiazepines.org.uk. Archived from the original on 8 December 2008. Retrieved 2008-10-31.

[112] "Discontinuation of Xanax" (PDF). Pfizer Australia.

[113] "DEA, Drug Scheduling". DEA. Archived from the original on 4 November 2008. Retrieved 2008-10-31.

[114] "Misuse of Drugs Act 1971 (c. 38)". The UK Statute Law database. 1991.

[115] British Medical Association, Royal Pharmaceutical Society of Great Britain (September 2010). "4.1.2: Anxiolytics". *British National Formulary (BNF 60)*. United Kingdom: BMJ Group and RPS Publishing. p. 212. ISBN 978-0-85369-931-6.

[116] "List of Psychotropic Substances under International Control" (PDF). *Incb.org*. International Narcotics Control Board. August 2003. Archived (PDF) from the original on 17 December 2008. Retrieved 2008-12-07.

[117] "Misuse Of Drugs (Amendment) Regulations". *Irish Statute Book*. Office of the Attorney General. 1993.

[118] "Läkemedelsverkets föreskrifter (LVFS 2011:10) om förteckningar över narkotika" [Medical Products Agency on the lists of drugs] (PDF) (in Swedish). Sweden: Läkemedelsverket. October 2011.

[119] "Alprazolam to be rescheduled from next year". 2013.

1.1.12 External links

- U.S. National Library of Medicine: Drug Information Portal – Alprazolam
- Erowid Alprazolam (Xanax) Vault

1.2 Benzodiazepine

Benzodiazepines (**BZD**), sometimes called "**benzos**", are a class of psychoactive drugs whose core chemical structure is the fusion of a benzene ring and a diazepine ring. The first such drug, chlordiazepoxide (Librium), was discovered accidentally by Leo Sternbach in 1955, and made available in 1960 by Hoffmann–La Roche - which, since 1963, has also marketed the benzodiazepine diazepam (Valium).[1] In 1977 benzodiazepines were globally the most prescribed medications.[2]

Benzodiazepines enhance the effect of the neurotransmitter gamma-aminobutyric acid (GABA) at the GABAA receptor, resulting in sedative, hypnotic (sleep-inducing), anxiolytic (anti-anxiety), anticonvulsant, and muscle relaxant properties. High doses of many shorter-acting benzodiazepines may also cause anterograde amnesia and dissociation.[3] These properties make benzodiazepines useful in treating anxiety, insomnia, agitation, seizures, muscle spasms, alcohol withdrawal and as a premedication for medical or dental procedures.[4] Benzodiazepines are categorized as either short-, intermediate-, or long-acting. Short- and intermediate-acting benzodiazepines are preferred for the treatment of insomnia; longer-acting benzodiazepines are recommended for the treatment of anxiety.[5]

Benzodiazepines are generally viewed as safe and effective for short-term use, although cognitive impairment and paradoxical effects such as aggression or behavioral disinhibition occasionally occur. A minority of people can have paradoxical reactions such as worsened agitation or panic.[6] Long-term use is controversial due to concerns about adverse psychological and physical effects, decreasing effectiveness, and physical dependence and withdrawal.[7][8] Due to adverse effects associated with the long-term use of benzodiazepines, withdrawal from benzodiazepines, in general, leads to improved physical and mental health.[9][10] The elderly are at an increased risk of suffering from both short- and long-term adverse effects,[9][11] and as a result all benzodiazepines are listed in the Beers List of inappropriate medications for older adults.[12]

There is controversy concerning the safety of benzodiazepines in pregnancy. While they are not major teratogens, uncertainty remains as to whether they cause cleft palate in a small number of babies and whether neurobehavioural effects occur as a result of prenatal exposure;[13] they are known to cause withdrawal symptoms in the newborn. Benzodiazepines can be taken in overdoses and can cause dangerous deep unconsciousness. However, they are much less toxic than their predecessors, the barbiturates, and death rarely results when a benzodiazepine is the only drug taken; however, when combined with other central nervous system (CNS) depressants such as ethanol and opioids, the potential for toxicity and fatal overdose increases.[14] Benzodiazepines are commonly misused and taken in combination with other drugs of abuse.[15][16][17]

1.2.1 Medical uses

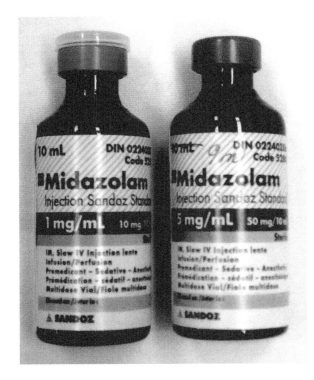

Midazolam 1 & 5 mg/mL injections (US)

See also: List of benzodiazepines

Benzodiazepines possess sedative, hypnotic, anxiolytic, anticonvulsant, muscle relaxant, and amnesic actions,[3][4] which are useful in a variety of indications such as alcohol dependence, seizures, anxiety, panic, agitation, and insomnia. Most are administered orally; however, they can also be given intravenously, intramuscularly, or rectally.[18]:189 In general, benzodiazepines are well-tolerated and are safe and effective drugs in the short term for a wide range of conditions.[19][20] Tolerance can develop to their effects and there is also a risk of dependence, and upon discontinuation a withdrawal syndrome may occur. These factors, combined with other possible secondary effects after prolonged use such as psychomotor, cognitive, or memory impairments, limit their long-term applicability.[21][22] The effects of long-term use or misuse include the tendency to cause or worsen cognitive deficits, depression, and anxiety.[9][11]

Panic disorder

Due to their effectiveness, tolerability, and rapid onset of anxiolytic action, benzodiazepines are frequently used for the treatment of anxiety associated with panic disorder.[23] However, there is disagreement among expert bodies regarding the long-term use of benzodiazepines for panic disorder. The views range from those that hold that benzodiazepines are not effective long-term [24] and that they should be reserved for treatment-resistant cases[25] to that they are as effective in the long term as selective serotonin reuptake inhibitors.[26]

The American Psychiatric Association (APA) guidelines[26] note that, in general, benzodiazepines are well tolerated, and their use for the initial treatment for panic disorder is strongly supported by numerous controlled trials. APA states that there is insufficient evidence to recommend any of the established panic disorder treatments over another. The choice of treatment between benzodiazepines, SSRIs, serotonin–norepinephrine reuptake inhibitors, tricyclic antidepressants, and psychotherapy should be based on the patient's history, preference, and other individual characteristics. Selective serotonin reuptake inhibitors are likely to be the best choice of pharmacotherapy for many patients with panic disorder, but benzodiazepines are also often used, and some studies suggest that these medications are still used with greater frequency than the SSRIs. One advantage of benzodiazepines is that they alleviate the anxiety symptoms much faster than antidepressants, and therefore may be preferred in patients for whom rapid symptom control is critical. However, this advantage is offset by the possibility of developing benzodiazepine dependence. APA does not recommend benzodiazepines for persons with depressive symptoms or a recent history of substance abuse. The APA guidelines state that, in general, pharmacotherapy of panic disorder should be continued for at least a year, and that clinical experience support continuing benzodiazepine treatment to prevent recurrence. Although major concerns about benzodiazepine tolerance and withdrawal have been raised, there is no evidence for significant dose escalation in patients using benzodiazepines long-term. For many such patients stable doses of benzodiazepines retain their efficacy over several years.[26]

Guidelines issued by the UK-based National Institute for Health and Clinical Excellence (NICE), carried out a systematic review using different methodology and came to a different conclusion. They questioned the accuracy of studies that were not placebo-controlled. And, based on the findings of placebo-controlled studies, they do not recommend use of benzodiazepines beyond two to four weeks, as tolerance and physical dependence develop rapidly, with withdrawal symptoms including rebound anxiety occurring after six weeks or more of use.[24][27] Nevertheless, benzodiazepines continue to be prescribed for the long-term treatment of anxiety disorders, although specific antidepressants and psychological therapies are recommended as the first-line treatment options with the anticonvulsant drug pregabalin indicated as a second- or third-line treatment and suitable for long-term use.[28] NICE stated that long-term use of benzodiazepines for panic disorder with or without agoraphobia is an unlicensed indication, does not have long-term efficacy, and is, therefore, not recommended by clinical guidelines. Psychological therapies such as cognitive behavioural therapy are recommended as a first-line therapy for panic disorder; benzodiazepine use has been found to interfere with therapeutic gains from these therapies.[24]

Benzodiazepines are usually administered orally; however, very occasionally lorazepam or diazepam may be given intravenously for the treatment of panic attacks.[18]

Generalized anxiety disorder

Benzodiazepines have robust efficacy in the short-term management of generalized anxiety disorder (GAD), but were not shown to be effective in producing long-term improvement overall.[29] According to National Institute for Health and Clinical Excellence (NICE), benzodiazepines can be used in the immediate management of GAD, if necessary. However, they should not usually be given for longer than 2–4 weeks. The only medications NICE recommends for the longer term management of GAD are antidepressants.[30]

Likewise, Canadian Psychiatric Association (CPA) recommends benzodiazepines alprazolam, bromazepam, lorazepam, and diazepam only as a second-line choice, if the treatment with two different antidepressants was unsuccessful. Although they are second-line agents, benzodiazepines can be used for a limited time to relieve severe anxiety and agitation. CPA guidelines note that after 4–6 weeks the effect of benzodiazepines may decrease to the level of placebo, and that benzodiazepines are less effective than antidepressants in alleviating ruminative worry, the core symptom of GAD. However, in some cases, a prolonged treatment with benzodiazepines as the add-on to an antidepressant may be justified.[31]

A 2015 review found a larger effect with medications than talk therapy.[32] Medications with benefit include serotonin-noradrenaline reuptake inhibitors, benzodiazepines, and selective serotonin reuptake inhibitors.[32]

Insomnia

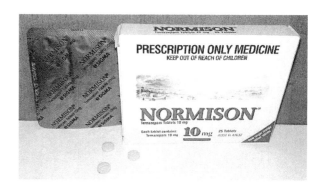

Temazepam (Normison) 10 mg tablets

Benzodiazepines can be useful for short-term treatment of insomnia. Their use beyond 2 to 4 weeks is not recommended due to the risk of dependence. It is preferred that benzodiazepines be taken intermittently and at the lowest effective dose. They improve sleep-related problems by shortening the time spent in bed before falling asleep, prolonging the sleep time, and, in general, reducing wakefulness.[33][34] However, they worsen sleep quality by increasing light sleep and decreasing deep sleep. Other drawbacks of hypnotics, including benzodiazepines, are possible tolerance to their effects, rebound insomnia, and reduced slow-wave sleep and a withdrawal period typified by rebound insomnia and a prolonged period of anxiety and agitation.[35][36]

The list of benzodiazepines approved for the treatment of insomnia is fairly similar among most countries, but which benzodiazepines are officially designated as first-line hypnotics prescribed for the treatment of insomnia can vary distinctly between countries.[34] Longer-acting benzodiazepines such as nitrazepam and diazepam have residual effects that may persist into the next day and are, in general, not recommended.[33]

It is not clear as to whether the new nonbenzodiazepine hypnotics (Z-drugs) are better than the short-acting benzodiazepines. The efficacy of these two groups of medications is similar.[33][36] According to the US Agency for Healthcare Research and Quality, indirect comparison indicates that side-effects from benzodiazepines may be about twice as frequent as from nonbenzodiazepines.[36] Some experts suggest using nonbenzodiazepines preferentially as a first-line long-term treatment of insomnia.[34] However, the UK National Institute for Health and Clinical Excellence did not find any convincing evidence in favor of Z-drugs. NICE review pointed out that short-acting Z-drugs were inappropriately compared in clinical trials with long-acting benzodiazepines. There have been no trials comparing short-acting Z-drugs with appropriate doses of short-acting benzodiazepines. Based on this, NICE recommended choosing the hypnotic based on cost and the patient's preference.[33]

Older adults should not use benzodiazepines to treat insomnia unless other treatments have failed to be effective.[37] When benzodiazepines are used, patients, their caretakers, and their physician should discuss the increased risk of harms, including evidence which shows twice the incidence of traffic collisions among driving patients as well as falls and hip fracture for all older patients.[37]

Seizures

Prolonged convulsive epileptic seizures are a medical emergency that can usually be dealt with effectively by administering fast-acting benzodiazepines, which are potent anticonvulsants. In a hospital environment, intravenous clonazepam, lorazepam, and diazepam are first-line choices, clonazepam due to its stronger and more potent anticonvulsant action, diazepam due to its faster onset and lorazepam for its longer duration of action. In the community, intravenous administration is not practical and so rectal diazepam or (more recently) buccal midazolam are used, with a preference for midazolam as its administration is easier and more socially acceptable.[38][39]

When benzodiazepines were first introduced, they were enthusiastically adopted for treating all forms of epilepsy. However, drowsiness and tolerance become problems with continued use and none are now considered first-line choices for long-term epilepsy therapy.[40] Clobazam is widely used by specialist epilepsy clinics worldwide and clonazepam is popular in the Netherlands, Belgium and France.[40] It was approved for use in the United States in 2011. In the UK, both clobazam and clonazepam are second-line choices for treating many forms of epilepsy.[41] Clobazam also has a useful role for very short-term seizure prophylaxis and in catamenial epilepsy.[40] Discontinuation after long-term use in epilepsy requires additional caution because of the risks of rebound seizures. Therefore, the dose is slowly tapered over a period of up to six months or longer.[39]

Alcohol withdrawal

Chlordiazepoxide is the most commonly used benzodiazepine for alcohol detoxification,[42] but diazepam may be used as an alternative. Both are used in the detoxification of individuals who are motivated to stop drinking, and are prescribed for a short period of time to reduce the risks of developing tolerance and dependence to the benzodiazepine medication itself.[18]:275 The benzodiazepines with a longer half-life make detoxification more tolerable, and dangerous (and potentially lethal) alcohol withdrawal effects are less likely to occur. On the other hand, short-acting benzodiazepines may lead to breakthrough seizures, and are, therefore, not recommended for detoxification in an outpatient setting. Oxazepam and lorazepam are often used in patients at risk of drug accumulation, in particular, the elderly and those with cirrhosis, because they are metabolized differently from other benzodiazepines, through conjugation.[43][44]

Benzodiazepines are the preferred choice in the management of alcohol withdrawal syndrome, in particular, for the prevention and treatment of the dangerous complication of seizures and in subduing severe delirium.[45] Lorazepam is the only benzodiazepine with predictable intramuscular absorption and it is the most effective in preventing and controlling acute seizures.[46]

Anxiety

Benzodiazepines are sometimes used in the treatment of acute anxiety, as they bring about rapid and marked or moderate relief of symptoms in most individuals;[24] however, they are not recommended beyond 2–4 weeks of use due to risks of tolerance and dependence and a lack of long-term effectiveness. As for insomnia, they may also be used on an irregular/"as-needed" basis, such as in cases where said anxiety is at its worst. Compared to other pharmacological treatments, benzodiazepines are twice as likely to lead to a relapse of the underlying condition upon discontinuation. Psychological therapies and other pharmacological therapies are recommended for the long-term treatment of generalized anxiety disorder. Antidepressants have higher remission rates and are, in general, safe and effective in the short and long term.[24]

Other indications

Benzodiazepines are often prescribed for a wide range of conditions:

- They can be very useful in intensive care to sedate patients receiving mechanical ventilation or those in extreme distress. Caution is exercised in this situation due to the occasional occurrence of respiratory depression, and it is recommended that benzodiazepine overdose treatment facilities should be available.[47]

- Benzodiazepines are effective as medication given a couple of hours before surgery to relieve anxiety. They also produce amnesia, which can be useful, as patients will not be able to remember any unpleasantness from the procedure.[48] They are also used in patients with dental phobia as well as some ophthalmic procedures like refractive surgery; although such use is controversial and only recommended for those who are very anxious.[49] Midazolam is the most commonly prescribed for this use because of its strong sedative actions and fast recovery time, as well as its water solubility, which reduces pain upon injection. Diazepam and lorazepam are sometimes used. Lorazepam has particularly marked amnesic properties that may make it more effective when amnesia is the desired effect.[18]:693

- Benzodiazepines are well known for their strong muscle-relaxing properties and can be useful in the treatment of muscle spasms,[18]:577–578 although tolerance often develops to their muscle relaxant effects.[9] Baclofen[50] or tizanidine are sometimes used as an alternative to benzodiazepines. Tizanidine has been found to have superior tolerability compared to diazepam and baclofen.[51]

- Benzodiazepines are also used to treat the acute panic caused by hallucinogen intoxication.[52] Benzodiazepines are also used to calm the acutely agitated individual and can, if required, be given via an intramuscular injection.[53] They can sometimes be effective in the short-term treatment of psychiatric emergencies such as acute psychosis as in schizophrenia or mania, bringing about rapid tranquillization and sedation until the effects of lithium or neuroleptics (antipsychotics) take effect. Lorazepam is most commonly used but clonazepam is sometimes prescribed for acute psychosis or mania;[54][55] their long-term use is not recommended due to risks of dependence.[18]:204

- Clonazepam, a benzodiazepine is used to treat many forms of parasomnia.[56] Rapid eye movement behavior disorder responds well to low doses of clonazepam.[57][58] Restless legs syndrome can be treated using clonazepam as a third line treatment option as the use of clonazepam is still investigational.[59][60]

- Benzodiazepines are sometimes used for obsessive compulsive disorder, although they are generally believed to be ineffective for this indication; effectiveness was, however, found in one small study.[61] Benzodiazepines can be considered as a treatment option in treatment resistant cases.[62]

- Antipsychotics are generally a first-line treatment for delirium; however, when delirium is caused by alcohol or sedative hypnotic withdrawal, benzodiazepines are a first-line treatment.[63]

- There is some evidence that low doses of benzodiazepines reduce adverse effects of electroconvulsive therapy.[64]

1.2.2 Adverse effects

See also: Long-term effects of benzodiazepines, Paradoxical reaction § Benzodiazepines and benzodiazepine withdrawal syndrome

The most common side-effects of benzodiazepines are related to their sedating and muscle-relaxing action. They include drowsiness, dizziness, and decreased alertness and concentration. Lack of coordination may result in falls and injuries, in particular, in the elderly.[65][66][67] Another result is impairment of driving skills and increased likelihood of road traffic accidents.[68][69] Decreased libido and erection problems are a common side effect. Depression and disinhibition may emerge. Hypotension and suppressed breathing (hypoventilation) may be encountered with intravenous use.[65][66] Less common side effects include nausea and changes in appetite, blurred vision, confusion, euphoria, depersonalization and nightmares. Cases of liver toxicity have been described but are very rare.[18]:183–189[70]

Paradoxical effects

Paradoxical reactions, such as increased seizures in epileptics,[71] aggression, violence, impulsivity, irritability and suicidal behavior sometimes occur. These reactions have been explained as consequences of disinhibition and the subsequent loss of control over socially unacceptable behavior. Paradoxical reactions are rare in the general population, with an incidence rate below 1% and similar to placebo.[6][72] However, they occur with greater frequency in recreational abusers, individuals with borderline personality disorder, children, and patients on high-dosage regimes.[73][74] In these groups, impulse control problems are perhaps the most important risk factor for disinhibition; learning disabilities and neurological disorders are also significant risks. Most reports of disinhibition involve high doses of high-potency benzodiazepines.[72]

Paradoxical effects may also appear after chronic use of benzodiazepines.[75]

Cognitive effects

The short-term use of benzodiazepines adversely affects multiple areas of cognition, the most notable one being that it interferes with the formation and consolidation of memories of new material and may induce complete anterograde amnesia.[65] However, researchers hold contrary opinions regarding the effects of long-term administration. One view is that many of the short-term effects continue into the long-term and may even worsen, and are not resolved after stopping benzodiazepine usage. Another view maintains that cognitive deficits in chronic benzodiazepine users occur only for a short period after the dose, or that the anxiety disorder is the cause of these deficits.

While the definitive studies are lacking, the former view received support from a 2004 meta-analysis of 13 small studies.[76][77] This meta-analysis found that long-term use of benzodiazepines was associated with moderate to large adverse effects on all areas of cognition, with visuospatial memory being the most commonly detected impairment. Some of the other impairments reported were decreased IQ, visiomotor coordination, information processing, verbal learning and concentration. The authors of the meta-analysis[76] and a later reviewer[77] noted that the applicability of this meta-analysis is limited because the subjects were taken mostly from withdrawal clinics; the coexisting drug, alcohol use, and psychiatric disorders were not defined; and several of the included studies conducted the cognitive measurements during the withdrawal period.

Long-term effects

The long-term effects of benzodiazepine use can include cognitive impairment as well as affective and behavioural problems. Feelings of turmoil, difficulty in thinking constructively, loss of sex-drive, agoraphobia and social phobia, increasing anxiety and depression, loss of interest in leisure pursuits and interests, and an inability to experience or express feelings can also occur. Not everyone, however, experiences problems with long-term use.[10][78] Additionally an altered perception of self, environment and relationships may occur.[77]

Withdrawal syndrome

Main articles: Benzodiazepine dependence, Benzodiazepine withdrawal syndrome and post-acute withdrawal syndrome

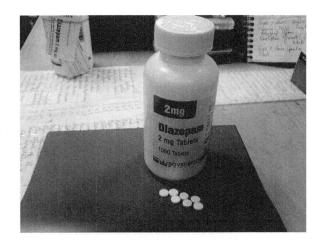

Diazepam 2 mg and 5 mg diazepam tablets, which are commonly used in the treatment of benzodiazepine withdrawal.

Tolerance, dependence and withdrawal The main problem of the chronic use of benzodiazepines is the development of tolerance and dependence. Tolerance manifests itself as diminished pharmacological effect and develops relatively quickly to the sedative, hypnotic, anticonvulsant, and muscle relaxant actions of benzodiazepines. Tolerance to anti-anxiety effects develops more slowly with little evidence of continued effectiveness beyond four to six months of continued use.[9] In general, tolerance to the amnesic effects does not occur.[79] However, controversy exists as to tolerance to the anxiolytic effects with some evidence that benzodiazepines retain efficacy[80] and opposing evidence from a systematic review of the literature that tolerance frequently occurs[19][24] and some evidence that anxiety may worsen with long-term use.[9] The question of tolerance to the amnesic effects of benzodiazepines is, likewise, unclear.[81] Some evidence suggests that partial tolerance does develop, and that, "memory impairment is limited to a narrow window within 90 minutes after each dose".[82]

Discontinuation of benzodiazepines or abrupt reduction of the dose, even after a relatively short course of treatment (three to four weeks), may result in two groups of symptoms — rebound and withdrawal. Rebound symptoms are the return of the symptoms for which the patient was treated but worse than before. Withdrawal symptoms are the new symptoms that occur when the benzodiazepine is stopped. They are the main sign of physical dependence.[82]

Withdrawal symptoms and management The most frequent symptoms of withdrawal from benzodiazepines are insomnia, gastric problems, tremors, agitation, fearfulness, and muscle spasms.[82] The less frequent effects are irritability, sweating, depersonalization, derealization, hypersensitivity to stimuli, depression, suicidal behavior, psychosis, seizures, and delirium tremens.[83] Severe symp-

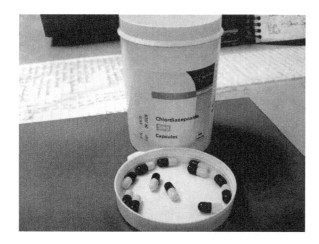

Chlordiazepoxide 5 mg capsules, which are sometimes used as an alternative to diazepam for benzodiazepine withdrawal. Like diazepam it has a long elimination half-life and long-acting active metabolites.

toms usually occur as a result of abrupt or over-rapid withdrawal. Abrupt withdrawal can be dangerous, therefore a gradual reduction regimen is recommended.[8]

Symptoms may also occur during a gradual dosage reduction, but are typically less severe and may persist as part of a protracted withdrawal syndrome for months after cessation of benzodiazepines.[84] Approximately 10% of patients will experience a notable protracted withdrawal syndrome, which can persist for many months or in some cases a year or longer. Protracted symptoms tend to resemble those seen during the first couple of months of withdrawal but usually are of a sub-acute level of severity. Such symptoms do gradually lessen over time, eventually disappearing altogether.[85]

Benzodiazepines have a reputation with patients and doctors for causing a severe and traumatic withdrawal; however, this is in large part due to the withdrawal process being poorly managed. Over-rapid withdrawal from benzodiazepines increases the severity of the withdrawal syndrome and increases the failure rate. A slow and gradual withdrawal customised to the individual and, if indicated, psychological support is the most effective way of managing the withdrawal. Opinion as to the time needed to complete withdrawal ranges from four weeks to several years. A goal of less than six months has been suggested,[8] but due to factors such as dosage and type of benzodiazepine, reasons for prescription, lifestyle, personality, environmental stresses, and amount of available support, a year or more may be needed to withdraw.[9][18]:183–184

Withdrawal is best managed by transferring the physically dependent patient to an equivalent dose of diazepam because it has the longest half-life of all of the benzodiazepines, is metabolised into long-acting active metabolites and is available in low-potency tablets, which can be quartered for smaller doses.[86] A further benefit is that it is available in liquid form, which allows for even smaller reductions.[8] Chlordiazepoxide, which also has a long half-life and long-acting active metabolites, can be used as an alternative.[86][87]

Nonbenzodiazepines are contraindicated during benzodiazepine withdrawal as they are cross tolerant with benzodiazepines and can induce dependence.[9] Alcohol is also cross tolerant with benzodiazepines and more toxic and thus caution is needed to avoid replacing one dependence with another.[86] During withdrawal, fluoroquinolone-based antibiotics are best avoided if possible; they displace benzodiazepines from their binding site and reduce GABA function and, thus, may aggravate withdrawal symptoms.[88] Antipsychotics are not recommended for benzodiazepine withdrawal (or other CNS depressant withdrawal states) especially clozapine, olanzapine or low potency phenothiazines e.g. chlorpromazine as they lower the seizure threshold and can worsen withdrawal effects; if used extreme caution is required.[89]

Withdrawal from long term benzodiazepines is beneficial for most individuals.[75] Withdrawal of benzodiazepines from long-term users, in general, leads to improved physical and mental health particularly in the elderly; although some long term users report continued benefit from taking benzodiazepines, this may be the result of suppression of withdrawal effects.[9][10]

1.2.3 Overdose

The use of flumazenil is controversial following benzodiazepine overdose.

Main article: Benzodiazepine overdose

Although benzodiazepines are much safer in overdose than their predecessors, the barbiturates, they can still cause problems in overdose.[14] Taken alone, they rarely cause severe complications in overdose;[90] statistics in England showed that benzodiazepines were responsible for 3.8% of all deaths by poisoning from a single drug.[15] However, combining these drugs with alcohol, opiates or tricyclic antidepressants markedly raises the toxicity.[16][91][92] The elderly are more sensitive to the side effects of benzodiazepines, and poisoning may even occur from their long-term use.[93] The various benzodiazepines differ in their toxicity; temazepam appears to be most toxic in overdose and when used with other drugs.[94][95] The symptoms of a benzodiazepine overdose may include; drowsiness, slurred speech, nystagmus, hypotension, ataxia, coma, respiratory depression, and cardiorespiratory arrest.[92]

A reversal agent for benzodiazepines exists, flumazenil (Anexate). Its use as an antidote is not routinely recommended due to the high risk of resedation and seizures.[96] In a double-blind, placebo-controlled trial of 326 patients, 4 patients suffered serious adverse events and 61% became resedated following the use of flumazenil.[97] Numerous contraindications to its use exist. It is contraindicated in patients with a history of long-term use of benzodiazepines, those having ingested a substance that lowers the seizure threshold or may cause an arrhythmia, and in those with abnormal vital signs.[98] One study found that only 10% of the patient population presenting with a benzodiazepine overdose are suitable candidates for treatment with flumazenil.[99]

1.2.4 Contraindications

Because of their muscle relaxant action, benzodiazepines may cause respiratory depression in susceptible individuals. For that reason, they are contraindicated in people with myasthenia gravis, sleep apnea, bronchitis, and COPD.[65][100] Caution is required when benzodiazepines are used in people with personality disorders or intellectual disability because of frequent paradoxical reactions.[65][100] In major depression, they may precipitate suicidal tendencies[101] and are sometimes used for suicidal overdoses.[100] Individuals with a history of alcohol, opioid and barbiturate abuse should avoid benzodiazepines, as there is a risk of life-threatening interactions with these drugs.[102]

Pregnancy

See also: Effects of benzodiazepines on newborns

In the United States, the Food and Drug Administration has categorized benzodiazepines into either category D or X meaning potential for harm in the unborn has been demonstrated.[103]

Exposure to benzodiazepines during pregnancy has been associated with a slightly increased (from 0.06 to 0.07%) risk of cleft palate in newborns, a controversial conclusion as some studies find no association between benzodiazepines and cleft palate. Their use by expectant mothers shortly before the delivery may result in a floppy infant syndrome, with the newborns suffering from hypotonia, hypothermia, lethargy, and breathing and feeding difficulties.[13][104] Cases of neonatal withdrawal syndrome have been described in infants chronically exposed to benzodiazepines in utero. This syndrome may be hard to recognize, as it starts several days after delivery, for example, as late as 21 day for chlordiazepoxide. The symptoms include tremors, hypertonia, hyperreflexia, hyperactivity, and vomiting and may last for up to three to six months.[13][105] Tapering down the dose during pregnancy may lessen its severity. If used in pregnancy, those benzodiazepines with a better and longer safety record, such as diazepam or chlordiazepoxide, are recommended over potentially more harmful benzodiazepines, such as temazepam[106] or triazolam. Using the lowest effective dose for the shortest period of time minimizes the risks to the unborn child.[107]

Elderly

The benefits of benzodiazepines are least and the risks are greatest in the elderly.[108][109] The elderly are at an increased risk of dependence and are more sensitive to the adverse effects such as memory problems, daytime sedation, impaired motor coordination, and increased risk of motor vehicle accidents and falls,[110] and an increased risk of hip fractures.[111] The long-term effects of benzodiazepines and benzodiazepine dependence in the elderly can resemble dementia, depression, or anxiety syndromes, and progressively worsens over time. Adverse effects on cognition can be mistaken for the effects of old age. The benefits of withdrawal include improved cognition, alertness, mobility, reduced risk incontinence, and a reduced risk of falls and fractures. The success of gradual-tapering benzodiazepines is as great in the elderly as in younger people. Benzodiazepines should be prescribed to the elderly only with caution and only for a short period at low doses.[112][113] Short to intermediate-acting benzodiazepines are preferred in the elderly such as oxazepam and temazepam. The high potency benzodiazepines alprazolam and triazolam and long-acting benzodiazepines are not recommended in the elderly due to increased adverse effects. Nonbenzodiazepines such as zaleplon and zolpidem and low doses of sedating antidepressants are sometimes used as alternatives to benzodiazepines.[113][114]

Long-term use of benzodiazepines has been associated with increased risk of cognitive impairment, but its relationship with dementia remains inconclusive.[115] The association of a past history of benzodiazepine use and cognitive decline is unclear, with some studies reporting a lower risk of cognitive decline in former users, some finding no association and some indicating an increased risk of cognitive decline.[116]

Benzodiazepines are sometimes prescribed to treat behavioral symptoms of dementia. However, like antidepressants, they have little evidence of effectiveness, although antipsychotics have shown some benefit.[117][118] Cognitive impairing effects of benzodiazepines that occur frequently in the elderly can also worsen dementia.[79]

1.2.5 Interactions

Individual benzodiazepines may have different interactions with certain drugs. Depending on their metabolism pathway, benzodiazepines can be divided roughly into two groups. The largest group consists of those that are metabolized by cytochrome P450 (CYP450) enzymes and possess significant potential for interactions with other drugs. The other group comprises those that are metabolized through glucuronidation, such as lorazepam, oxazepam, and temazepam, and, in general, have few drug interactions.[100]

Many drugs, including oral contraceptives, some antibiotics, antidepressants, and antifungal agents, inhibit cytochrome enzymes in the liver. They reduce the rate of elimination of the benzodiazepines that are metabolized by CYP450, leading to possibly excessive drug accumulation and increased side-effects. In contrast, drugs that induce cytochrome P450 enzymes, such as St John's wort, the antibiotic rifampicin, and the anticonvulsants carbamazepine and phenytoin, accelerate elimination of many benzodiazepines and decrease their action.[102][119] Taking benzodiazepines with alcohol, opioids and other central nervous system depressants potentiates their action. This often results in increased sedation, impaired motor coordination, suppressed breathing, and other adverse effects that have potential to be lethal.[102][119] Antacids can slow down absorption of some benzodiazepines; however, this effect is marginal and inconsistent.[102]

1.2.6 Pharmacology

Benzodiazepines share a similar chemical structure, and their effects in humans are mainly produced by the allosteric modification of a specific kind of neurotransmitter receptor, the GABAA receptor, which increases the overall conductance of these inhibitory channels; this results in the various therapeutic effects as well as adverse effects of benzodiazepines.[120] Other less important mechanisms of action are also known.[121][122]

Common types

- 2-keto compounds:

    chlordiazepoxide, clorazepate, diazepam, flurazepam, halazepam, prazepam, and others.[123][124]

- 3-hydroxy compounds:

    lorazepam, lormetazepam, oxazepam, temazepam[123][124]

- 7-nitro compounds:

    clonazepam, flunitrazepam, nimetazepam, nitrazepam[123][124]

- Triazolo compounds:

    adinazolam, alprazolam, estazolam, triazolam[123][124]

- Imidazo compounds

    climazolam, loprazolam, midazolam[123][124]

Chemistry

Left: The 1,4-benzodiazepine ring system. *Right*: 5-phenyl-1H-benzo[e] [1,4]diazepin-2(3H)-one forms the skeleton of many of the most common benzodiazepine pharmaceuticals, such as diazepam (7-chloro-1-methyl substituted).

The term *benzodiazepine* is the chemical name for the heterocyclic ring system (see figure to the right), which is a fusion between the benzene and diazepine ring systems.[126]

1.2. BENZODIAZEPINE

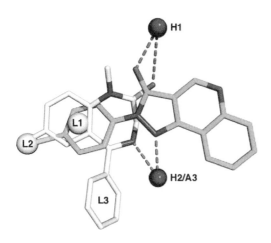

A pharmacophore model of the benzodiazepine binding site on the GABAA receptor.[125] White sticks represent the carbon atoms of the benzodiazepine diazepam, while green represents carbon atoms of the nonbenzodiazepine CGS-9896. Red and blue sticks are oxygen and nitrogen atoms that are present in both structures. The red spheres labeled H1 and H2/A3 are, respectively, hydrogen bond donating and accepting sites in the receptor, while L1, L2, and L3 denote lipophilic binding sites.

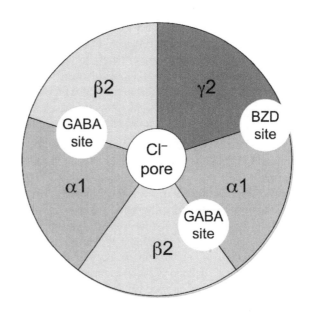

Schematic diagram of the $(\alpha 1)_2(\beta 2)_2(\gamma 2)$ GABAA receptor complex that depicts the five-protein subunits that form the receptor, the chloride (Cl^-) ion channel pore at the center, the two GABA active binding sites at the $\alpha 1$ and $\beta 2$ interfaces and the benzodiazepine (BZD) allosteric binding site at the $\alpha 1$ and $\gamma 2$ interface.

Under Hantzsch–Widman nomenclature, a diazepine is a heterocycle with two nitrogen atoms, five carbon atom and the maximum possible number of cumulative double bonds. The "benzo" prefix indicates the benzene ring fused onto the diazepine ring.[126]

Benzodiazepine drugs are substituted 1,4-benzodiazepines, although the chemical term can refer to many other compounds that do not have useful pharmacological properties. Different benzodiazepine drugs have different side groups attached to this central structure. The different side groups affect the binding of the molecule to the GABAA receptor and so modulate the pharmacological properties.[120] Many of the pharmacologically active "classical" benzodiazepine drugs contain the 5-phenyl-1H-benzo[e] [1,4]diazepin-2(3H)-one substructure (see figure to the right).[127] Benzodiazepines have been found to mimic protein reverse turns structurally which enable them with their biological activity in many cases.,[128][129]

Nonbenzodiazepines also bind to the benzodiazepine binding site on the GABAA receptor and possess similar pharmacological properties. While the nonbenzodiazepines are by definition structurally unrelated to the benzodiazepines, both classes of drugs possess a common pharmacophore (see figure to the lower-right), which explains their binding to a common receptor site.[125]

Mechanism of action

Benzodiazepines work by increasing the efficiency of a natural brain chemical, GABA, to decrease the excitability of neurons. This reduces the communication between neurons and, therefore, has a calming effect on many of the functions of the brain.

GABA controls the excitability of neurons by binding to the GABAA receptor.[120] The GABAA receptor is a protein complex located in the synapses of neurons. All GABAA receptors contain an ion channel that conducts chloride ions across neuronal cell membranes and two binding sites for the neurotransmitter gamma-aminobutyric acid (GABA), while a subset of GABAA receptor complexes also contain a single binding site for benzodiazepines. Binding of benzodiazepines to this receptor complex does not alter binding of GABA. Unlike other positive allosteric modulators that increases ligand binding, benzodiazepine binding acts as a positive allosteric modulator by increasing the total conduction of chloride ions across the neuronal cell membrane when GABA is already bound to its receptor. This increased chloride ion influx hyperpolarizes the neuron's membrane potential. As a result, the difference between resting potential and threshold potential is increased and firing is less likely. Different GABAA receptor subtypes have varying distributions within different regions of the brain and, therefore, control distinct neuronal circuits. Hence, activation of different GABAA receptor subtypes by benzodiazepines may result in distinct pharmacological actions.[130] In terms of the mechanism of action of benzodiazepines, their similarities are too great to separate them into individual categories such as anxiolytic or hypnotic. For example, a hypnotic administered in low doses will produce anxiety-relieving effects, whereas a benzodiazepine marketed as an anti-anxiety drug will at higher doses induce sleep.[131]

The subset of GABAA receptors that also bind benzodiazepines are referred to as benzodiazepine receptors (BzR). The GABAA receptor is a heteromer composed of five subunits, the most common ones being two αs, two βs, and one γ ($\alpha_2\beta_2\gamma$). For each subunit, many subtypes exist (α_{1-6}, β_{1-3}, and γ_{1-3}). GABAA receptors that are made up of different combinations of subunit subtypes have different properties, different distributions in the brain and different activities relative to pharmacological and clinical effects.[132] Benzodiazepines bind at the interface of the α and γ subunits on the GABAA receptor. Binding also requires that alpha subunits contain a histidine amino acid residue, (i.e., α_1, α_2, α_3, and α_5 containing GABAA receptors). For this reason, benzodiazepines show no affinity for GABAA receptors containing α_4 and α_6 subunits with an arginine instead of a histidine residue.[133] Once bound to the benzodiazepine receptor, the benzodiazepine ligand locks the benzodiazepine receptor into a conformation in which it has a greater affinity for the GABA neurotransmitter. This increases the frequency of the opening of the associated chloride ion channel and hyperpolarizes the membrane of the associated neuron. The inhibitory effect of the available GABA is potentiated, leading to sedatory and anxiolytic effects. For instance, those ligands with high activity at the α_1 are associated with stronger hypnotic effects, whereas those with higher affinity for GABAA receptors containing α_2 and/or α_3 subunits have good anti-anxiety activity.[134]

The benzodiazepine class of drugs also interact with peripheral benzodiazepine receptors. Peripheral benzodiazepine receptors are present in peripheral nervous system tissues, glial cells, and to a lesser extent the central nervous system.[135] These peripheral receptors are not structurally related or coupled to GABAA receptors. They modulate the immune system and are involved in the body response to injury.[121][136] Benzodiazepines also function as weak adenosine reuptake inhibitors. It has been suggested that some of their anticonvulsant, anxiolytic, and muscle relaxant effects may be in part mediated by this action.[122]

1.2.7 Pharmacokinetics

A benzodiazepine can be placed into one of three groups by its elimination half-life, or time it takes for the body to eliminate half of the dose.[138] Some benzodiazepines have long-acting active metabolites, such as diazepam and chlordiazepoxide, which are metabolised into desmethyldiazepam. Desmethyldiazepam has a half-life of 36–200 hours, and flurazepam, with the main active metabolite of desalkylflurazepam, with a half-life of 40–250 hours. These long-acting metabolites are partial agonists.[5][86]

- Short-acting compounds have a median half-life of 1–12 hours. They have few residual effects if taken before bedtime, rebound insomnia may occur upon discontinuation, and they might cause daytime withdrawal symptoms such as next day rebound anxiety with prolonged usage. Examples are brotizolam, midazolam, and triazolam.

- Intermediate-acting compounds have a median half-life of 12–40 hours. They may have some residual effects in the first half of the day if used as a hypnotic. Rebound insomnia, however, is more common upon discontinuation of intermediate-acting benzodiazepines than longer-acting benzodiazepines. Examples are alprazolam, estazolam, flunitrazepam, clonazepam, lormetazepam, lorazepam, nitrazepam, and temazepam.

- Long-acting compounds have a half-life of 40–250 hours. They have a risk of accumulation in the elderly and in individuals with severely impaired liver function, but they have a reduced severity of rebound effects and withdrawal. Examples are diazepam, clorazepate, chlordiazepoxide, and flurazepam.

1.2.8 History

The first benzodiazepine, chlordiazepoxide (*Librium*), was synthesized in 1955 by Leo Sternbach while working at Hoffmann–La Roche on the development of tranquilizers. The pharmacological properties of the compounds prepared initially were disappointing, and Sternbach abandoned the project. Two years later, in April 1957, co-worker Earl Reeder noticed a "nicely crystalline" compound left over from the discontinued project while spring-cleaning in the lab. This compound, later named chlordiazepoxide, had not been tested in 1955 because of Sternbach's focus on other issues. Expecting the pharmacology results to be negative and hoping to publish the chemistry-related findings, researchers submitted it for a standard battery of animal tests. However, the compound showed very strong sedative, anticonvulsant, and muscle relaxant effects. These impressive clinical findings led to its speedy introduction throughout the world in 1960 under the brand name *Librium*.[139][140] Following chlordiazepoxide, diazepam marketed by Hoffmann–La Roche under the

The molecular structure of chlordiazepoxide, the first benzodiazepine. It was marketed by Hoffmann–La Roche from 1960 branded as Librium.

brand name *Valium* in 1963, and for a while the two were the most commercially successful drugs. The introduction of benzodiazepines led to a decrease in the prescription of barbiturates, and by the 1970s they had largely replaced the older drugs for sedative and hypnotic uses.[1]

The new group of drugs was initially greeted with optimism by the medical profession, but gradually concerns arose; in particular, the risk of dependence became evident in the 1980s. Benzodiazepines have a unique history in that they were responsible for the largest-ever class-action lawsuit against drug manufacturers in the United Kingdom, involving 14,000 patients and 1,800 law firms that alleged the manufacturers knew of the dependence potential but intentionally withheld this information from doctors. At the same time, 117 general practitioners and 50 health authorities were sued by patients to recover damages for the harmful effects of dependence and withdrawal. This led some doctors to require a signed consent form from their patients and to recommend that all patients be adequately warned of the risks of dependence and withdrawal before starting treatment with benzodiazepines.[141] The court case against the drug manufacturers never reached a verdict; legal aid had been withdrawn and there were allegations that the consultant psychiatrists, the expert witnesses, had a conflict of interest. This litigation led to changes in the British law, making class action lawsuits more difficult.[142]

Although antidepressants with anxiolytic properties have been introduced, and there is increasing awareness of the adverse effects of benzodiazepines, prescriptions for short-term anxiety relief have not significantly dropped.[7] For treatment of insomnia, benzodiazepines are now less popular than nonbenzodiazepines, which include zolpidem, zaleplon and eszopiclone.[143] Nonbenzodiazepines are molecularly distinct, but nonetheless, they work on the same benzodiazepine receptors and produce similar sedative effects.[144]

1.2.9 Recreational use

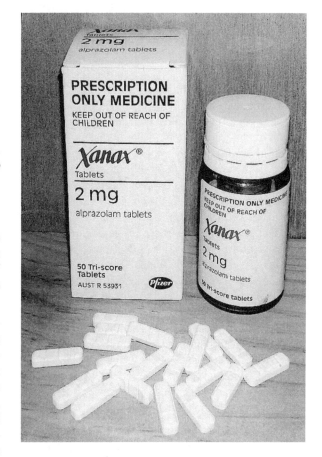

Xanax (alprazolam) 2 mg tri-score tablets

Main articles: Benzodiazepine drug misuse and Drug-related crime

Benzodiazepines are considered to be major drugs of abuse.[17] Benzodiazepine abuse is mostly limited to individuals who abuse other drugs, i.e., poly-drug abusers. On the international scene, benzodiazepines are categorized as Schedule IV controlled drugs by the INCB, apart from flunitrazepam which is a Schedule III drug under the Convention on Psychotropic Substances.[145] Some variation in drug scheduling exists in individual countries; for example, in the United Kingdom, midazolam and temazepam are Schedule III controlled drugs. British law requires temazepam (but *not* midazolam) to be stored in safe custody. Safe custody requirements ensures that pharmacists and doctors holding stock of temazepam must store it in securely fixed double-locked steel safety cabinets and maintain a written register, which must be bound and contain separate entries for temazepam and must be written in ink with no use of correction fluid (although a written register is not required for temazepam in the United Kingdom). Disposal of expired stock must be witnessed by a designated inspector (either a local drug-enforcement police officer or official from health authority).[146][147] Benzodiazepine abuse ranges from occasional binges on large doses, to chronic and compulsive drug abuse of high doses.[148]

Benzodiazepines are used recreationally and by problematic drug misusers. Mortality is higher among poly-drug misusers that also use benzodiazepines. Heavy alcohol use also increases mortality among poly-drug users.[15] Dependence and tolerance, often coupled with dosage escalation, to benzodiazepines can develop rapidly among drug misusers; withdrawal syndrome may appear after as little as three weeks of continuous use. Long-term use has the potential to cause both physical and psychological dependence and severe withdrawal symptoms such as depression, anxiety (often to the point of panic attacks), and agoraphobia.[11] Benzodiazepines and, in particular, temazepam are sometimes used intravenously, which, if done incorrectly or in an unsterile manner, can lead to medical complications including abscesses, cellulitis, thrombophlebitis, arterial puncture, deep vein thrombosis, and gangrene. Sharing syringes and needles for this purpose also brings up the possibility of transmission of hepatitis, HIV, and other diseases. Benzodiazepines are also misused intranasally, which may have additional health consequences. Once benzodiazepine dependence has been established, a clinician usually converts the patient to an equivalent dose of diazepam before beginning a gradual reduction program.[149]

A 1999–2005 Australian police survey of detainees reported preliminary findings that self-reported users of benzodiazepines were less likely than non-user detainees to work full-time and more likely to receive government benefits, use methamphetamine or heroin, and be arrested or imprisoned.[150] Benzodiazepines are sometimes used for criminal purposes; they serve to incapacitate a victim in cases of drug assisted rape or robbery.[151]

Overall, anecdotal evidence suggests that temazepam may be the most psychologically habit-forming (addictive) benzodiazepine. Temazepam abuse reached epidemic proportions in some parts of the world, in particular, in Europe and Australia, and is a major drug of abuse in many Southeast Asian countries. This led authorities of various countries to place temazepam under a more restrictive legal status. Some countries, such as Sweden, banned the drug outright.[152] Temazepam also has certain pharmacokinetic properties of absorption, distribution, elimination, and clearance that make it more apt to abuse compared to many other benzodiazepines.[153][154]

1.2.10 Veterinary use

Benzodiazepines are used in veterinary practice in the treatment of various disorders and conditions. As in humans, they are used in the first-line management of seizures, status epilepticus, and tetanus, and as maintenance therapy in epilepsy (in particular, in cats).[155][156][157] They are widely used in small and large animals (including horses, swine, cattle and exotic and wild animals) for their anxiolytic and sedative effects, as pre-medication before surgery, for induction of anesthesia and as adjuncts to anesthesia.[155][158]

1.2.11 References

[1] Shorter E (2005). "Benzodiazepines". *A Historical Dictionary of Psychiatry*. Oxford University Press. pp. 41–2. ISBN 0-19-517668-5.

[2] *Treating Alcohol and Drug Problems in Psychotherapy Practice Doing What Works*. New York: Guilford Publications. 2011. p. 47. ISBN 9781462504381.

[3] Page C, Michael C, Sutter M, Walker M, Hoffman BB (2002). *Integrated Pharmacology* (2nd ed.). C.V. Mosby. ISBN 978-0-7234-3221-0.

[4] Olkkola KT, Ahonen J (2008). "Midazolam and other benzodiazepines". *Handb Exp Pharmacol*. Handbook of Experimental Pharmacology **182** (182): 335–60. doi:10.1007/978-3-540-74806-9_16. ISBN 978-3-540-72813-9. PMID 18175099.

[5] Dikeos DG, Theleritis CG, Soldatos CR (2008). "Benzodiazepines: effects on sleep". In Pandi-Perumal SR, Verster JC, Monti JM, Lader M, Langer SZ (eds.). *Sleep Disorders: Diagnosis and Therapeutics*. Informa Healthcare. pp. 220–2. ISBN 0-415-43818-7.

[6] Saïas T, Gallarda T (2008). "[Paradoxical aggressive reactions to benzodiazepine use: a review]". *Encephale* (in French) **34** (4): 330–6. doi:10.1016/j.encep.2007.05.005. PMID 18922233.

[7] Lader M (2008). "Effectiveness of benzodiazepines: do they work or not?". *Expert Rev Neurother* (PDF) **8** (8): 1189–91. doi:10.1586/14737175.8.8.1189. PMID 18671662.

[8] Lader M, Tylee A, Donoghue J (2009). "Withdrawing benzodiazepines in primary care". *CNS Drugs* **23** (1): 19–34. doi:10.2165/0023210-200923010-00002. PMID 19062773.

[9] Ashton H (2005). "The diagnosis and management of benzodiazepine dependence" (PDF).

Current Opinion in Psychiatry **18** (3): 249–55. doi:10.1097/01.yco.0000165594.60434.84. PMID 16639148.

[10] Ashton H (2004). "Benzodiazepine dependence". In Haddad P, Dursun S, Deakin B (eds.). *Adverse Syndromes and Psychiatric Drugs: A Clinical Guide*. Oxford University Press. pp. 239–60. ISBN 978-0-19-852748-0.

[11] McIntosh A, Semple D, Smyth R, Burns J, Darjee R (2005). "Depressants". *Oxford Handbook of Psychiatry* (1st ed.). Oxford University Press. p. 540. ISBN 0-19-852783-7.

[12] American Geriatrics Society 2012 Beers Criteria Update Expert Panel (2012). "American Geriatrics Society updated Beers Criteria for potentially inappropriate medication use in older adults" (PDF). U.S. Department of Health & Human Services. *guideline.gov*. Agency for Healthcare Research and Quality.

[13] American College of Obstetricians and Gynecologists Committee on Practice Bulletins—Obstetrics (April 2008). "ACOG Practice Bulletin no. 92: Use of psychiatric medications during pregnancy and lactation". *Obstet Gynecol* **111** (4): 1001–20. doi:10.1097/AOG.0b013e31816fd910. PMID 18378767. Lay summary.

[14] Fraser AD (1998). "Use and abuse of the benzodiazepines". *Ther Drug Monit* **20** (5): 481–9. doi:10.1097/00007691-199810000-00007. PMID 9780123.

[15] Charlson F, Degenhardt L, McLaren J, Hall W, Lynskey M (2009). "A systematic review of research examining benzodiazepine-related mortality". *Pharmacoepidemiol Drug Saf* **18** (2): 93–103. doi:10.1002/pds.1694. PMID 19125401.

[16] White JM, Irvine RJ (1999). "Mechanisms of fatal opioid overdose". *Addiction* **94** (7): 961–72. doi:10.1046/j.1360-0443.1999.9479612.x. PMID 10707430.

[17] Lader MH (1999). "Limitations on the use of benzodiazepines in anxiety and insomnia: are they justified?". *Eur Neuropsychopharmacol* **9** (Suppl 6): S399–405. doi:10.1016/S0924-977X(99)00051-6. PMID 10622686.

[18] Royal Pharmaceutical Society of Great Britain (2009). *British National Formulary (BNF 57)*. BMJ Group and RPS Publishing. ISBN 978-0-85369-845-6.

[19] Perugi G, Frare F, Toni C (2007). "Diagnosis and treatment of agoraphobia with panic disorder". *CNS Drugs* **21** (9): 741–64. doi:10.2165/00023210-200721090-00004. PMID 17696574.

[20] Tesar GE (1990). "High-potency benzodiazepines for short-term management of panic disorder: the U.S. experience". *J Clin Psychiatry* **51** (Suppl): 4–10; discussion 50–3. PMID 1970816.

[21] Faught E (2004). "Treatment of refractory primary generalized epilepsy". *Rev Neurol Dis* **1** (Suppl 1): S34–43. PMID 16400293.

[22] Allgulander C, Bandelow B, Hollander E, Montgomery SA, Nutt DJ, Okasha A, Pollack MH, Stein DJ, Swinson RP (2003). "WCA recommendations for the long-term treatment of generalized anxiety disorder". *CNS Spectr* **8** (Suppl 1): 53–61. PMID 14767398.

[23] Stevens JC, Pollack MH (2005). "Benzodiazepines in clinical practice: consideration of their long-term use and alternative agents". *Journal of Clinical Psychiatry* **66** (Suppl 2): 21–27. PMID 15762816. The frequent use of benzodiazepines for the treatment of anxiety is likely a reflection of their effectiveness, rapid onset of anxiolytic effect, and tolerability.

[24] McIntosh A, Cohen A, Turnbull N; et al. (2004). "Clinical guidelines and evidence review for panic disorder and generalised anxiety disorder" (PDF). National Collaborating Centre for Primary Care. Retrieved 2009-06-16.

[25] Bandelow B, Zohar J, Hollander E, Kasper S, Möller HJ (October 2002). "World Federation of Societies of Biological Psychiatry (WFSBP) Guidelines for the Pharmacological Treatment of Anxiety, Obsessive-Compulsive and Posttraumatic Stress Disorders". *The World Journal of Biological Psychiatry* (Informa Healthcare) **3** (4): 171–99. doi:10.3109/15622970209150621. PMID 12516310.

[26] Work Group on Panic Disorder (January 2009). "APA Practice Guideline for the Treatment of Patients With Panic Disorder, Second Edition" (PDF). Retrieved July 12, 2009.

[27] Barbui C, Cipriani A (2009). "Proposal for the inclusion in the WHO Model List of Essential Medicines of a selective serotonin-reuptake inhibitor for Generalised Anxiety Disorder" (PDF). WHO Collaborating Centre for Research and Training in Mental Health. Retrieved 2009-06-23.

[28] Cloos JM, Ferreira V (2009). "Current use of benzodiazepines in anxiety disorders". *Current Opinion in Psychiatry* **22** (1): 90–95. doi:10.1097/YCO.0b013e32831a473d. PMID 19122540.

[29] Martin JL, Sainz-Pardo M, Furukawa TA, Martín-Sánchez E, Seoane T, Galán C (September 2007). "Benzodiazepines in generalized anxiety disorder: heterogeneity of outcomes based on a systematic review and meta-analysis of clinical trials". *J. Psychopharmacol. (Oxford)* **21** (7): 774–82. doi:10.1177/0269881107077355. PMID 17881433.

[30] "Clinical Guideline 22 (amended). Anxiety: management of anxiety (panic disorder, with or without agoraphobia, and generalised anxiety disorder) in adults in primary, secondary and community care" (PDF). National Institute for Health and Clinical Excellence. 2007. pp. 23–25. Retrieved 2009-08-08.

[31] Canadian Psychiatric Association (July 2006). "Clinical practice guidelines. Management of anxiety disorders". *Can J Psychiatry* (PDF) **51** (8 Suppl 2): 51S–55S. PMID 16933543. Retrieved 2009-08-08.

[32] Bandelow B, Reitt M, Röver C, Michaelis S, Görlich Y, Wedekind D (2015). "Efficacy of treatments for anxiety disorders: a meta-analysis". *International Clinical Psychopharmacology* **30** (4): 183–92. doi:10.1097/YIC.0000000000000078. PMID 25932596.

[33] "Technology Appraisal Guidance 77. Guidance on the use of zaleplon, zolpidem and zopiclone for the short-term management of insomnia" (PDF). National Institute for Clinical Excellence. April 2004. Retrieved 2009-07-26.

[34] Ramakrishnan K, Scheid DC (August 2007). "Treatment options for insomnia". *American Family Physician* **76** (4): 517–26. PMID 17853625.

[35] Carlstedt RA (13 December 2009). *Handbook of Integrative Clinical Psychology, Psychiatry, and Behavioral Medicine: Perspectives, Practices, and Research*. Springer Publishing Company. pp. 128–30. ISBN 0-8261-1094-0.

[36] Buscemi N, Vandermeer B, Friesen C, Bialy L, Tubman M, Ospina M, Klassen TP, Witmans M (June 2005). "Manifestations and Management of Chronic Insomnia in Adults. Summary, Evidence Report/Technology Assessment: Number 125" (PDF). Agency for Healthcare Research and Quality.

[37] American Geriatrics Society. "Five Things Physicians and Patients Should Question". *Choosing Wisely: an initiative of the ABIM Foundation* (American Geriatrics Society). Retrieved August 1, 2013, which cites

- Finkle WD, Der JS, Greenland S, Adams JL, Ridgeway G, Blaschke T, Wang Z, Dell RM, VanRiper KB (2011). "Risk of Fractures Requiring Hospitalization After an Initial Prescription for Zolpidem, Alprazolam, Lorazepam, or Diazepam in Older Adults". *Journal of the American Geriatrics Society* **59** (10): 1883–1890. doi:10.1111/j.1532-5415.2011.03591.x. PMID 22091502.

- Allain H, Bentué-Ferrer D, Polard E, Akwa Y, Patat A (2005). "Postural instability and consequent falls and hip fractures associated with use of hypnotics in the elderly: A comparative review". *Drugs & aging* **22** (9): 749–765. doi:10.2165/00002512-200522090-00004. PMID 16156679.

- "American Geriatrics Society Updated Beers Criteria for Potentially Inappropriate Medication Use in Older Adults". *Journal of the American Geriatrics Society* **60** (4): 616–631. 2012. doi:10.1111/j.1532-5415.2012.03923.x. PMC 3571677. PMID 22376048.

[38] Scottish Intercollegiate Guidelines Network (2005). "Diagnosis and management of epilepsy in adults" (PDF). pp. 17–9. Retrieved 2009-06-05.

[39] Stokes T, Shaw EJ, Juarez-Garcia A, Camosso-Stefinovic J, Baker R (October 2004). *Clinical Guidelines and Evidence Review for the Epilepsies: diagnosis and management in adults and children in primary and secondary care* (PDF). London: Royal College of General Practitioners. pp. 61, 64–65. Retrieved 2009-06-02.

[40] Shorvon SD (March 2009). "Drug treatment of epilepsy in the century of the ILAE: the second 50 years, 1959–2009". *Epilepsia* **50** (Suppl 3): 93–130. doi:10.1111/j.1528-1167.2009.02042.x. PMID 19298435.

[41] Stokes T, Shaw EJ, Juarez-Garcia A, Camosso-Stefinovic J, Baker R (October 2004). "Clinical Guidelines and Evidence Review for the Epilepsies: diagnosis and management in adults and children in primary and secondary care (Appendix B)" (PDF). London: Royal College of General Practitioners. p. 432. Retrieved 2009-06-02.

[42] Ashworth M, Gerada C (1997). "ABC of mental health. Addiction and dependence—II: Alcohol". *BMJ* **315** (7104): 358–60. doi:10.1136/bmj.315.7104.358. PMC 2127236. PMID 9270461.

[43] Kraemer KL, Conigliaro J, Saitz R (1999). "Managing alcohol withdrawal in the elderly". *Drugs Aging* **14** (6): 409–25. doi:10.2165/00002512-199914060-00002. PMID 10408740.

[44] Prater CD, Miller KE, Zylstra RG (September 1999). "Outpatient detoxification of the addicted or alcoholic patient". *American Family Physician* **60** (4): 1175–83. PMID 10507746.

[45] Ebell MH (April 2006). "Benzodiazepines for alcohol withdrawal". *American Family Physician* **73** (7): 1191. PMID 16623205.

[46] Peppers MP (1996). "Benzodiazepines for alcohol withdrawal in the elderly and in patients with liver disease". *Pharmacotherapy* **16** (1): 49–57. PMID 8700792.

[47] Devlin JW, Roberts RJ (July 2009). "Pharmacology of commonly used analgesics and sedatives in the ICU: benzodiazepines, propofol, and opioids". *Crit Care Clin* **25** (3): 431–49, vii. doi:10.1016/j.ccc.2009.03.003. PMID 19576523.

[48] Broscheit J, Kranke P (February 2008). "[The preoperative medication: background and specific indications for the selection of the drugs]". *Anasthesiol Intensivmed Notfallmed Schmerzther* **43** (2): 134–43. doi:10.1055/s-2008-1060547. PMID 18293248.

[49] Berthold C (May 2007). "Enteral sedation: safety, efficacy, and controversy". *Compend Contin Educ Dent* **28** (5): 264–71; quiz 272, 282. PMID 17607891.

[50] Mañon-Espaillat R, Mandel S (1999). "Diagnostic algorithms for neuromuscular diseases". *Clin Podiatr Med Surg* **16** (1): 67–79. PMID 9929772.

[51] Kamen L, Henney HR, Runyan JD (February 2008). "A practical overview of tizanidine use for spasticity secondary to multiple sclerosis, stroke, and spinal cord injury". *Curr Med Res Opin* **24** (2): 425–39. doi:10.1185/030079908X261113. PMID 18167175.

[52] Wyatt JP, Illingworth RN, Robertson CE, Clancy MJ, Munro PT (2005). "Poisoning". *Oxford Handbook of Accident and Emergency Medicine* (2nd ed.). Oxford University Press. pp. 173–208. ISBN 978-0-19-852623-0.

[53] Zimbroff DL (2008). "Pharmacological control of acute agitation: focus on intramuscular preparations". *CNS Drugs* **22** (3): 199–212. doi:10.2165/00023210-200822030-00002. PMID 18278976.

[54] Curtin F, Schulz P (2004). "Clonazepam and lorazepam in acute mania: a Bayesian meta-analysis". *J Affect Disord* **78** (3): 201–8. doi:10.1016/S0165-0327(02)00317-8. PMID 15013244.

[55] Gillies D, Beck A, McCloud A, Rathbone J, Gillies D (2005). Gillies, Donna, ed. "Benzodiazepines alone or in combination with antipsychotic drugs for acute psychosis". *Cochrane Database of Systematic Reviews* (4): CD003079. doi:10.1002/14651858.CD003079.pub2. PMID 16235313.

[56] Schenck CH, Arnulf I, Mahowald MW (June 2007). "Sleep and Sex: What Can Go Wrong? A Review of the Literature on Sleep Related Disorders and Abnormal Sexual Behaviors and Experiences". *Sleep* **30** (6): 683–702. PMC 1978350. PMID 17580590.

[57] Ferini-Strambi L, Zucconi M (September 2000). "REM sleep behavior disorder". *Clin Neurophysiol.* 111 Suppl 2: S136–40. doi:10.1016/S1388-2457(00)00414-4. PMID 10996567.

[58] Silber MH (February 2001). "Sleep disorders". *Neurol Clin* **19** (1): 173–86. doi:10.1016/S0733-8619(05)70011-6. PMID 11471763.

[59] Grupo Brasileiro de Estudos em Síndrome das Pernas Inquietas (GBE-SPI) (September 2007). "Síndrome das pernas inquietas: diagnóstico e tratamento. Opinião de especialistas brasileiros" [Restless legs syndrome: diagnosis and treatment. Opinion of Brazilian experts]. *Arq. Neuro-Psiquiatr.* (in Portuguese) **65** (3a): 721–7. doi:10.1590/S0004-282X2007000400035. ISSN 0004-282X. PMID 17876423.

[60] Trenkwalder C, Hening WA, Montagna P, Oertel WH, Allen RP, Walters AS, Costa J, Stiasny-Kolster K, Sampaio C (December 2008). "Treatment of restless legs syndrome: an evidence-based review and implications for clinical practice" (PDF). *Mov Disord* **23** (16): 2267–302. doi:10.1002/mds.22254. PMID 18925578.

[61] Schatzberg AF, Nemeroff CB, eds. (May 6, 2009). *The American Psychiatric Publishing Textbook of Psychopharmacology* (Fourth ed.). American Psychiatric Publishing. p. 470. ISBN 978-1-58562-309-9.

[62] Bandelow B (September 2008). "The medical treatment of obsessive-compulsive disorder and anxiety". *CNS Spectr* **13** (9 Suppl 14): 37–46. PMID 18849910.

[63] Attard A, Ranjith G, Taylor D (August 2008). "Delirium and its treatment". *CNS Drugs* **22** (8): 631–44. doi:10.2165/00023210-200822080-00002. PMID 18601302.

[64] Gallegos J, Vaidya P, D'Agati D, Jayaram G, Nguyen T, Tripathi A, Trivedi JK, Reti IM (June 2012). "Decreasing adverse outcomes of unmodified electroconvulsive therapy: suggestions and possibilities". *J ECT* **28** (2): 77–81. doi:10.1097/YCT.0b013e3182359314. PMID 22531198.

[65] Ballenger JC (2000). "Benzodiazepine receptors agonists and antagonists". In Sadock VA, Sadock BJ, Kaplan HI (eds.). *Kaplan & Sadock's Comprehensive Textbook of Psychiatry* (7th ed.). Lippincott Williams & Wilkins. pp. 2317–23. ISBN 0-683-30128-4.

[66] Tasman A, Lieberman JA (2006). *Handbook of Psychiatric Drugs*. Wiley. p. 151. ISBN 0-470-02821-1.

[67] Stone KL, Ensrud KE, Ancoli-Israel S (September 2008). "Sleep, insomnia and falls in elderly patients". *Sleep Med.* 9 Suppl 1: S18–22. doi:10.1016/S1389-9457(08)70012-1. PMID 18929314.

[68] Rapoport MJ, Lanctôt KL, Streiner DL, Bédard M, Vingilis E, Murray B, Schaffer A, Shulman KI, Herrmann N (2009). "Benzodiazepine use and driving: a meta-analysis". *J Clin Psychiatry* **70** (5): 663–73. doi:10.4088/JCP.08m04325. PMID 19389334.

[69] Orriols L, Salmi LR, Philip P, Moore N, Delorme B, Castot A, Lagarde E (2009). "The impact of medicinal drugs on traffic safety: a systematic review of epidemiological studies". *Pharmacoepidemiol Drug Saf* **18** (8): 647–58. doi:10.1002/pds.1763. PMC 2780583. PMID 19418468.

[70] *"benzodiazepines-oral"* at medicinenet.com

[71] Riss J, Cloyd J, Gates J, Collins S (August 2008). "Benzodiazepines in epilepsy: pharmacology and pharmacokinetics". *Acta Neurol Scand* **118** (2): 69–86. doi:10.1111/j.1600-0404.2008.01004.x. PMID 18384456.

[72] Paton C (2002). "Benzodiazepines and disinhibition: a review" (PDF). *Psychiatr Bull R Coll Psychiatr* **26** (12): 460–2. doi:10.1192/pb.26.12.460.

[73] Bond AJ (1998). "Drug-induced behavioural disinhibition: incidence, mechanisms and therapeutic implications". *CNS Drugs* **9** (1): 41–57. doi:10.2165/00023210-199809010-00005.

[74] Drummer OH (2002). "Benzodiazepines—effects on human performance and behavior". *Forensic Sci Rev* **14** (1–2): 1–14.

[75] Ashton H (2007). "Drug dependency: benzodiazepines". In Ayers S, Baum A, McManus C, Newman S (eds.). *Cambridge Handbook of Psychology, Health and Medicine* (2nd ed.). Cambridge University Press. pp. 675–8. ISBN 978-0-521-87997-2.

[76] Barker MJ, Greenwood KM, Jackson M, Crowe SF (2004). "Cognitive effects of long-term benzodiazepine use: a meta-analysis". *CNS Drugs* **18** (1): 37–48. doi:10.2165/00023210-200418010-00004. PMID 14731058.

[77] Stewart SA (2005). "The effects of benzodiazepines on cognition" (PDF). *J Clin Psychiatry* **66** (Suppl 2): 9–13. PMID 15762814.

[78] Hammersley D, Beeley L (1996). "The effects of medication on counselling". In Palmer S, Dainow S, Milner P. *Counselling: The BACP Counselling Reader* **1**. Sage. pp. 211–4. ISBN 978-0-8039-7477-7.

[79] Longo LP, Johnson B (April 2000). "Addiction: Part I. Benzodiazepines—side effects, abuse risk and alternatives". *American Family Physician* **61** (7): 2121–8. PMID 10779253.

[80] Nardi AE, Perna G (May 2006). "Clonazepam in the treatment of psychiatric disorders: an update". *Int Clin Psychopharmacol* **21** (3): 131–42. doi:10.1097/01.yic.0000194379.65460.a6. PMID 16528135.

[81] Otto MW, Bruce SE, Deckersbach T (2005). "Benzodiazepine use, cognitive impairment, and cognitive-behavioral therapy for anxiety disorders: issues in the treatment of a patient in need" (PDF). *J Clin Psychiatry* **66** (Suppl 2): 34–8. PMID 15762818.

[82] Chouinard G (2004). "Issues in the clinical use of benzodiazepines: potency, withdrawal, and rebound" (PDF). *J Clin Psychiatry* **65** (Suppl 5): 7–12. PMID 15078112.

[83] Harrison PC, Gelder MG, Cowen P (2006). "The misuse of alcohol and drugs". *Shorter Oxford Textbook of Psychiatry* (5th ed.). Oxford University Press. pp. 461–2. ISBN 0-19-856667-0.

[84] Judith Collier, Murray Longmore, Keith Amarakone (31 January 2013). "Psychiatry". *Oxford Handbook of Clinical Specialties*. OUP Oxford. p. 368. ISBN 978-0-19-150476-1.

[85] Ashton H (1991). "Protracted withdrawal syndromes from benzodiazepines". *J Subst Abuse Treat* **8** (1–2): 19–28. doi:10.1016/0740-5472(91)90023-4. PMID 1675688.

[86] Ashton CH (2002). *Benzodiazepines: how they work & how to withdraw (aka The Ashton Manual)*. Retrieved 2009-05-27.

[87] Lal R, Gupta S, Rao R, Kattimani S (2007). "Emergency management of substance overdose and withdrawal" (PDF). *Substance Use Disorder*. World Health Organization (WHO). p. 82. Retrieved 2009-06-06. Generally, a longer-acting benzodiazepine such as chlordiazepoxide or diazepam is used and the initial dose titrated downward

[88] Ford C, Law F (July 2014). "Guidance for the use and reduction of misuse of benzodiazepines and other hypnotics and anxiolytics in general practice" (PDF). *smmgp.org.uk*.

[89] Ebadi M (23 October 2007). "Alphabetical presentation of drugs". *Desk Reference for Clinical Pharmacology* (2nd ed.). USA: CRC Press. p. 512. ISBN 978-1-4200-4743-1.

[90] Gaudreault P, Guay J, Thivierge RL, Verdy I (1991). "Benzodiazepine poisoning. Clinical and pharmacological considerations and treatment". *Drug Saf* **6** (4): 247–65. doi:10.2165/00002018-199106040-00003. PMID 1888441.

[91] Robin Mantooth (28 January 2010). "Toxicity, benzodiazepine". *eMedicine*. Retrieved 2010-10-02.

[92] Ramrakha P, Moore K (2004). "Chapter 14: Drug overdoses". *Oxford Handbook of Acute Medicine* (2nd ed.). Oxford University Press. pp. 791–838 (798). ISBN 0-19-852072-7.

[93] Klein-Schwartz W, Oderda GM (1991). "Poisoning in the elderly. Epidemiological, clinical and management considerations". *Drugs Aging* **1** (1): 67–89. doi:10.2165/00002512-199101010-00008. PMID 1794007.

[94] Buckley NA, Dawson AH, Whyte IM, O'Connell DL (1995). "Relative toxicity of benzodiazepines in overdose". *BMJ* **310** (28): 219–221. doi:10.1136/bmj.310.6974.219. PMC 2548618. PMID 7866122.

[95] Serfaty M, Masterton G (1994). "Fatal poisonings attributed to benzodiazepines in Britain during the 1980s". *British Journal of Psychiatry* **163** (1): 128–9. doi:10.1192/bjp.163.3.386. PMID 8104653.

[96] Seger DL (2004). "Flumazenil—treatment or toxin". *J Toxicol Clin Toxicol* **42** (2): 209–16. doi:10.1081/CLT-120030946. PMID 15214628.

[97] "Treatment of benzodiazepine overdose with flumazenil. The flumazenil in benzodiazepine intoxication multicenter study group". *Clin Ther* **14** (6): 978–95. 1992. PMID 1286503.

[98] Spivey WH (1992). "Flumazenil and seizures: analysis of 43 cases". *Clin Ther* **14** (2): 292–305. PMID 1611650.

[99] Goldfrank LR (2002). *Goldfrank's Toxicologic Emergencies*. McGraw-Hill. ISBN 0-07-136001-8.

[100] Meyler L, Aronson JK, ed. (2006). *Meyler's Side Effects of Drugs: the International Encyclopedia of Adverse Drug Reactions and Interactions* (15th ed.). Elsevier. pp. 429–43. ISBN 0-444-50998-4.

[101] Committee on Safety of Medicines (1988). "Benzodiazepines, dependence and withdrawal symptoms" (PDF). Medicines and Healthcare products Regulatory Agency. Retrieved 2009-05-28.

[102] Moody D (2004). "Drug interactions with benzodiazepines". In Raymon LP, Mozayani A (eds.). *Handbook of Drug Interactions: a Clinical and Forensic Guide*. Humana. pp. 3–88. ISBN 1-58829-211-8.

[103] Roach SS, Ford SM (2006). "Sedatives and hypnotics". *Introductory Clinical Pharmacology* (8th ed.). Lippincott Williams & Wilkins. p. 236. ISBN 978-0-7817-7595-3.

[104] Dolovich LR, Addis A, Vaillancourt JM, Power JD, Koren G, Einarson TR (September 1998). "Benzodiazepine use in pregnancy and major malformations or oral cleft: meta-analysis of cohort and case-control studies" (PDF). *BMJ* **317** (7162): 839–43. doi:10.1136/bmj.317.7162.839. PMC 31092. PMID 9748174.

[105] American Academy of Pediatrics Committee on Drugs (1998). "Neonatal drug withdrawal" (PDF). *Pediatrics* **101** (6): 1079–88. PMID 9614425.

[106] Temazepam-Rxlist Pregnancy Category@

[107] Iqbal MM, Sobhan T, Ryals T (2002). "Effects of commonly used benzodiazepines on the fetus, the neonate and the nursing infant" (PDF). *Psychiatr Serv* **53** (1): 39–49. doi:10.1176/appi.ps.53.1.39. PMID 11773648.

[108] Tariq SH, Pulisetty S (2008). "Pharmacotherapy for insomnia". *Clin Geriatr Med* **24** (1): 93–105, vii. doi:10.1016/j.cger.2007.08.009. PMID 18035234.

[109] Bain KT (2006). "Management of chronic insomnia in elderly persons". *Am J Geriatr Pharmacother* **4** (2): 168–92. doi:10.1016/j.amjopharm.2006.06.006. PMID 16860264.

[110] Allain H, Bentué-Ferrer D, Polard E, Akwa Y, Patat A (2005). "Postural instability and consequent falls and hip fractures associated with use of hypnotics in the elderly: a comparative review". *Drugs Aging* **22** (9): 749–65. doi:10.2165/00002512-200522090-00004. PMID 16156679.

[111] Khong TP, de Vries F, Goldenberg JS, Klungel OH, Robinson NJ, Ibáñez L, Petri H (July 2012). "Potential impact of benzodiazepine use on the rate of hip fractures in five large European countries and the United States". *Calcif. Tissue Int.* **91** (1): 24–31. doi:10.1007/s00223-012-9603-8. PMC 3382650. PMID 22566242.

[112] Bogunovic OJ, Greenfield SF (2004). "Practical geriatrics: Use of benzodiazepines among elderly patients" (PDF). *Psychiatr Serv* **55** (3): 233–5. doi:10.1176/appi.ps.55.3.233. PMID 15001721.

[113] Jackson SG, Jansen P, Mangoni A (22 May 2009). *Prescribing for Elderly Patients*. Wiley. pp. 47–48. ISBN 0-470-02428-3.

[114] Rosenthal TC, Williams M, Naughton BJ (2006). *Office care geriatrics*. Philadelphia: Lippincott Williams Wilkins. pp. 260–262. ISBN 0-7817-6196-4.

[115] Hulse GK, Lautenschlager NT, Tait RJ, Almeida OP (2005). "Dementia associated with alcohol and other drug use". *Int Psychogeriatr* **17** (Suppl 1): S109–27. doi:10.1017/S1041610205001985. PMID 16240487.

[116] Verdoux H, Lagnaoui R, Begaud B (2005). "Is benzodiazepine use a risk factor for cognitive decline and dementia? A literature review of epidemiological studies". *Psychol Med* **35** (3): 307–15. doi:10.1017/S0033291704003897. PMID 15841867.

[117] Snowden M, Sato K, Roy-Byrne P (2003). "Assessment and treatment of nursing home residents with depression or behavioral symptoms associated with dementia: a review of the literature". *J Am Geriatr Soc* **51** (9): 1305–17. doi:10.1046/j.1532-5415.2003.51417.x. PMID 12919245.

[118] Wang PS, Brookhart MA, Setoguchi S, Patrick AR, Schneeweiss S (2006). "Psychotropic medication use for behavioral symptoms of dementia". *Curr Neurol Neurosci Rep* **6** (6): 490–5. doi:10.1007/s11910-006-0051-6. PMID 17074284.

[119] Norman TR, Ellen SR, Burrows GD (1997). "Benzodiazepines in anxiety disorders: managing therapeutics and dependence" (PDF). *Med J Aust* **167** (9): 490–5. PMID 9397065.

[120] Olsen RW, Betz H (2006). "GABA and glycine". In Siegel GJ, Albers RW, Brady S, Price DD (eds.). *Basic Neurochemistry: Molecular, Cellular and Medical Aspects* (7th ed.). Elsevier. pp. 291–302. ISBN 0-12-088397-X.

[121] Zavala F (1997). "Benzodiazepines, anxiety and immunity". *Pharmacol Ther* **75** (3): 199–216. doi:10.1016/S0163-7258(97)00055-7. PMID 9504140.

[122] Narimatsu E, Niiya T, Kawamata M, Namiki A (2006). "[The mechanisms of depression by benzodiazepines, barbiturates and propofol of excitatory synaptic transmissions mediated by adenosine neuromodulation]". *Masui* (in Japanese) **55** (6): 684–91. PMID 16780077.

[123] Juergens, MD, Steven M. "Understanding Benzodiazepines" (PDF). California Society of Addiction Medicine. Retrieved 25 April 2012.

[124] Carlo P, Finollo R, Ledda A, Brambilla G (January 1989). "Absence of liver DNA fragmentation in rats treated with high oral doses of 32 benzodiazepine drugs". *Fundamental and Applied Toxicology* **12** (1): 34–41. doi:10.1016/0272-0590(89)90059-6. PMID 2925017.

[125] Madsen U, Bräuner-Osborne H, Greenwood JR, Johansen TN, Krogsgaard-Larsen P, Liljefors T, Nielsen M, Frølund B (2005). "GABA and Glutamate receptor ligands and their therapeutic potential in CNS disorders". In Gad SC. *Drug Discovery Handbook*. Hoboken, N.J: Wiley-Interscience/J. Wiley. pp. 797–907. ISBN 0-471-21384-5.

[126] Panico R, Powell WH, Richer JC, eds. (1993). *A Guide to IUPAC Nomenclature of Organic Compounds*.

IUPAC/Blackwell Science. pp. 40–3. ISBN 0-632-03488-2.; Moss GP (1998). "Nomenclature of fused and bridged fused ring systems (IUPAC Recommendations 1998)" (PDF). *Pure Appl Chem* **70** (1): 143–216. doi:10.1351/pac199870010143.

[127] CAS registry number:2898-08-0 1,3-dihydro-5-phenyl-2H-1,4-benzodiazepin-2-one; other names: Ro 05-2921, dechlorodemethyldiazepam.

[128] Ripka WC, De Lucca GV, Bach AC, Pottorf RS, Blaney JM (1993). "Protein β-turn mimetics I. Design, synthesis, and evaluation in model cyclic peptides". *Tetrahedron* **49** (17): 3593–3608. doi:10.1016/S0040-4020(01)90217-0.

[129] Hata M, Marshall GR (2006). "Do benzodiazepines mimic reverse-turn structures?". *Journal of Computer-Aided Molecular Design* **20** (5): 321–331. doi:10.1007/s10822-006-9059-x. PMID 16972167.

[130] Rudolph U, Möhler H (2006). "GABA-based therapeutic approaches: GABAA receptor subtype functions". *Current Opinion in Pharmacology* **6** (1): 18–23. doi:10.1016/j.coph.2005.10.003. PMID 16376150.

[131] Puri BK, Tyrer P (28 August 1998). "Clinical psychopharmacology". *Sciences Basic to Psychiatry* (2nd ed.). Churchill Livingstone. pp. 155–156. ISBN 978-0-443-05514-0. Retrieved 11 July 2009.

[132] Johnston GA (1996). "GABAA receptor pharmacology". *Pharmacol Ther* **69** (3): 173–98. doi:10.1016/0163-7258(95)02043-8. PMID 8783370.

[133] Wafford KA, Macaulay AJ, Fradley R, O'Meara GF, Reynolds DS, Rosahl TW (2004). "Differentiating the role of gamma-aminobutyric acid type A (GABAA) receptor subtypes". *Biochem Soc Trans* **32** (Pt3): 553–6. doi:10.1042/BST0320553. PMID 15157182.

[134] Hevers W, Lüddens H (1998). "The diversity of GABAA receptors. Pharmacological and electrophysiological properties of GABAA channel subtypes". *Mol Neurobiol* **18** (1): 35–86. doi:10.1007/BF02741459. PMID 9824848.

[135] Arvat E, Giordano R, Grottoli S, Ghigo E (2002). "Benzodiazepines and anterior pituitary function". *J Endocrinol Invest* **25** (8): 735–47. doi:10.1007/bf03345110. PMID 12240908.

[136] Zisterer DM, Williams DC (1997). "Peripheral-type benzodiazepine receptors". *Gen Pharmacol* **29** (3): 305–14. doi:10.1016/S0306-3623(96)00473-9. PMID 9378234.

[137] O'Brien (2005). "Benzodiazepine Use, Abuse, and Dependence" (PDF). *J Clin Psychiatry*: 66. Retrieved 5 September 2013.

[138] Cardinali DP, Monti JM (2006). "Chronopharmacology and its implication to the pharmacology of sleep". In Pandi-Perumal SR, Monti JM. *Clinical pharmacology of sleep*. Basel: Birkhäuser. pp. 211–3. ISBN 9783764374402.

[139] Sternbach LH (1979). "The benzodiazepine story". *Journal of Medicinal Chemistry* **22** (1): 1–7. doi:10.1021/jm00187a001. PMID 34039. During this cleanup operation, my co-worker, Earl Reeder, drew my attention to a few hundred milligrams of two products, a nicely crystalline base and its hydrochloride. Both the base, which had been prepared by treating the quinazoline N-oxide 11 with methylamine, and its hydrochloride had been made sometime in 1955. The products were not submitted for pharmacological testing at that time because of our involvement with other problems

[140] Miller NS, Gold MS (1990). "Benzodiazepines: reconsidered". *Adv Alcohol Subst Abuse* **8** (3–4): 67–84. doi:10.1300/J251v08n03_06. PMID 1971487.

[141] King MB (1992). "Is there still a role for benzodiazepines in general practice?". *Br J Gen Pract* **42** (358): 202–5. PMC 1372025. PMID 1389432.

[142] Peart R (1999-06-01). "Memorandum by Dr Reg Peart". *Minutes of Evidence*. Select Committee on Health, House of Commons, UK Parliament. Retrieved 2009-05-27.

[143] Jufe GS (Jul–Aug 2007). "[New hypnotics: perspectives from sleep physiology]". *Vertex* **18** (74): 294–9. PMID 18265473.

[144] Lemmer B (2007). "The sleep–wake cycle and sleeping pills". *Physiol Behav* **90** (2–3): 285–93. doi:10.1016/j.physbeh.2006.09.006. PMID 17049955.

[145] International Narcotics Control Board (2003). "List of psychotropic substances under international control" (PDF). Retrieved 2008-12-17.

[146] Home Office (2005). Explanatory memorandum to the misuse of drugs and the misuse of drugs (supply to addicts) (amendment) regulations 2005.No.2864. Accessed 20–10–03

[147] "List of drugs currently controlled under the misuse of drugs legislation" (PDF). UK Government Home Office. 2010-10-25. Retrieved 2011-01-30.

[148] Karch SB (20 December 2006). *Drug Abuse Handbook* (2nd ed.). United States of America: CRC Press. p. 217. ISBN 978-0-8493-1690-6.

[149] Gerada C, Ashworth M (1997). "ABC of mental health. Addiction and dependence—I: Illicit drugs". *BMJ* **315** (7103): 297–300. doi:10.1136/bmj.315.7103.297. PMC 2127199. PMID 9274553.

[150] Loxley W (2007). "Benzodiazepine use and harms among police detainees in Australia" (PDF). *Trends Issues Crime Crim Justice* (Canberra, A.C.T.: Australian Institute of Criminology) (336). ISSN 0817-8542. Retrieved 2009-06-10.

[151] Kintz P (2007). "Bioanalytical procedures for detection of chemical agents in hair in the case of drug-facilitated crimes". *Anal Bioanal Chem* **388** (7): 1467–74. doi:10.1007/s00216-007-1209-z. PMID 17340077.

[152] "Benzodiazepine abuse". Benzo.org.uk. Retrieved 2011-11-28.

[153] Farré M, Camí J (December 1991). "Pharmacokinetic considerations in abuse liability evaluation". *Br J Addict.* **86** (12): 1601–6. doi:10.1111/j.1360-0443.1991.tb01754.x. PMID 1786493.

[154] Busto U, Sellers EM (1986). "Pharmacokinetic determinants of drug abuse and dependence. A conceptual perspective". *Clin Pharmacokinet.* **11** (2): 144–153. doi:10.2165/00003088-198611020-00004. PMID 3514044.

[155] Kahn CM, Line S, Aiello SE, ed. (2005). *The Merck Veterinary Manual* (9th ed.). Wiley. ISBN 978-0-911910-50-6.

[156] Frey HH (1989). "Anticonvulsant drugs used in the treatment of epilepsy". *Probl Vet Med* **1** (4): 558–77. PMID 2520134.

[157] Podell M (1996). "Seizures in dogs". *Vet Clin North Am Small Anim Pract* **26** (4): 779–809. PMID 8813750.

[158] Gross ME (2001). "Tranquilizers, α$_2$-adrenergic agonists, and related agents". In Adams RH (ed.). *Veterinary Pharmacology and Therapeutics* (8th ed.). Iowa State University Press. pp. 325–33. ISBN 0-8138-1743-9.

1.2.12 External links

- National Institute on Drug Abuse: "NIDA for Teens: Prescription Depressant Medications".* Ashton CH (2002). *Benzodiazepines: how they work & how to withdraw (aka The Ashton Manual). The Ashton Manual.* Retrieved 2009-06-09.

- Ashton CH (2007). "Benzodiazepine equivalence table". Retrieved 2009-06-09.

- Fruchtengarten L (April 1998). Ruse M, ed. "Benzodiazepines". *Poisons Information Monograph (Group monograph) G008.* IPCS INCHEM. Retrieved 2009-06-09.

- Longo LP, Johnson B (April 2000). "Addiction: Part I. Benzodiazepines—side effects, abuse risk and alternatives". *American Family Physician* **61** (7): 2121–8. PMID 10779253.

- "The complete story of the benzodiazepines". The Eaton T. Fores Research Center. 2005. Archived from the original on June 5, 2009. Retrieved 2009-06-09.

- "Benzodiazepines". Drugs.com.

- Benzodiazepines – information from mental health charity The Royal College of Psychiatrists

- "Benzodiazepines". RxList.

- *"benzodiazepines-oral"* at medicinenet.com

1.3 Anxiolytic

An **anxiolytic** (also **antipanic** or **antianxiety agent**)[1] is a medication or other intervention that inhibits anxiety. This effect is in contrast to anxiogenic agents, which increase anxiety. Together these categories of psychoactive compounds or interventions may be referred to as anxiotropic compounds/agents. Some recreational drugs such as ethanol (alcohol) induce anxiolysis initially, however studies show that many of these drugs are anxiogenic. Anxiolytic medications have been used for the treatment of anxiety and its related psychological and physical symptoms. Anxiolytics have been shown to be useful in the treatment of anxiety disorders. Light therapy and other interventions have also been found to have an anxiolytic effect.[2]

Beta-receptor blockers such as propranolol and oxprenolol, although not anxiolytics, can be used to combat the somatic symptoms of anxiety, as tachycardia and palpitations.[3]

Anxiolytics are also known as **minor tranquilizers**.[4] The term is less common in modern texts, and was originally derived from a dichotomy with major tranquilizers, also known as neuroleptics or antipsychotics.

1.3.1 Alternatives to medication

Psychotherapeutic treatment can be an effective alternative to medication.[5] Exposure therapy is the recommended treatment for phobic anxiety disorders. Cognitive behavioral therapy (CBT) has been found to be effective treatment for panic disorder, social anxiety disorder, generalized anxiety disorder, and obsessive-compulsive disorder. Healthcare providers can also help by educating sufferers about anxiety disorders and referring individuals to self-help resources.[6] CBT has been shown to be effective in the treatment of generalized anxiety disorder, and possibly more effective than pharmacological treatments in the long term.[7] Sometimes medication is combined with psychotherapy, but research has not found a benefit of combined pharmacotherapy and psychotherapy versus monotherapy.[8]

However, even with CBT being a viable treatment option, it can still be ineffective for many individuals. Both the Canadian and American medical associations then suggest the use of a strong but long lasting benzodiazepine such as clonazepam and alprazolam and an antidepressant, usually Prozac for its effectiveness.[9]

Note that adolescent anxiety once the patient becomes pubescent can often turn into depression, at which time other treatments may be required.

1.3.2 Medications

Barbiturates

Main article: Barbiturate

Barbiturates exert an anxiolytic effect linked to the sedation they cause. The risk of abuse and addiction is high. Many experts consider these drugs obsolete for treating anxiety but valuable for the short-term treatment of severe insomnia, though only after benzodiazepines or non-benzodiazepines have failed.

Benzodiazepines

Main article: Benzodiazepine

Benzodiazepines are prescribed for short-term relief of severe and disabling anxiety. Benzodiazepines may also be indicated to cover the latent periods associated with the medications prescribed to treat an underlying anxiety disorder. They are used to treat a wide variety of conditions and symptoms and are usually a first choice when short-term CNS sedation is needed. Longer-term uses include treatment for severe anxiety. If benzodiazepines are discontinued rapidly after being taken daily for two or more weeks there is a risk of benzodiazepine withdrawal and rebound syndrome, and tolerance and dependence may also occur, but may be clinically acceptable.[10] There is also the added problem of the accumulation of drug metabolites and adverse effects.[11] Benzodiazepines include:

- Alprazolam (Xanax)
- Bromazepam (Lectopam, Lexotan)
- Chlordiazepoxide (Librium)
- Clonazepam (Klonopin, Rivotril)
- Clorazepate (Tranxene)
- Diazepam (Valium)
- Flurazepam (Dalmane)
- Lorazepam (Ativan)
- Oxazepam (Serax, Serapax)
- Temazepam (Restoril)
- Triazolam (Halcion)

Benzodiazepines exert their anxiolytic properties at moderate dosage. At higher dosage hypnotic properties occur.[12]

- Tofisopam (Emandaxin and Grandaxin) is a drug that is a benzodiazepine derivative. Like other benzodiazepines, it possesses anxiolytic properties, but, unlike other benzodiazepines, it does not have anticonvulsant, sedative, skeletal muscle relaxant, motor skill-impairing, or amnestic properties.

Antidepressants

Serotonergic antidepressants Selective serotonin reuptake inhibitors or **serotonin-specific reuptake inhibitor**[13] (**SSRIs**) are a class of compounds typically used as antidepressants in the treatment of depression, anxiety disorders, and some personality disorders. SSRIs are primarily classified as antidepressants and typically higher dosages are required to be effective against anxiety disorders than to be effective against depression; nevertheless, most SSRIs have anxiolytic properties. They can, however, be anxiogenic early on in the course of treatment due to negative feedback through the serotonergic autoreceptors. For this reason in some individuals a low dose concurrent benzodiazepine therapy might be beneficial during the early stages of serotonergic therapy to counteract the initial anxiogenic effects current serotonergics antidepressants have.

Serotonin–norepinephrine reuptake inhibitor Serotonin–norepinephrine reuptake inhibitor include venlafaxine and duloxetine drugs. Venlafaxine, in extended release form, and duloxetine, are indicated for the treatment of GAD. SSNRIs are as effective as SSRIs in the treatment of anxiety disorders.[14]

Tricyclic antidepressant Older tricyclic antidepressants (TCAs) are anxiolytic too; however, their side effects are often more severe in nature. Examples include imipramine, doxepin, amitriptyline, and the unrelated trazodone.

Tetracyclic antidepressant Mirtazapine has demonstrated anxiolytic effects with a better side effect profile to all other classes of antidepressants, for example it rarely causes or exacerbates anxiety. However, it in many countries (such as USA and Australia) it is not specifically approved for anxiety disorders and is only used off label.

Monoamine oxidase inhibitors Monoamine oxidase inhibitors (MAOIs) are very effective for anxiety, but due to drug dangers, are rarely prescribed. Examples include: phenelzine, isocarboxazid and tranylcypromine. A reversible MAOI, which has none of the dietary restrictions associated with classic MAOI's, moclobemide is used in Canada and the UK as 'Manerix' and in Australia as 'Aurorix' which have none of the more severe SSRI's and SNRI's caused SSRI discontinuation syndrome, an often overlooked and damaging syndrome which is objectively and subjectively as bad or, for some, even worse than Benzodiazepine withdrawal syndrome.

Beta blockers

Although not officially approved for this purpose, Beta blockers also can have an antianxiety effect.[15][16]

Miscellaneous

Alpha-adrenergic agonist   Alpha 2A receptor agonists Clonidine and Guanfacine has demonstrated both anxiolytic and anxiogenic effects.

Mebicar   Mebicar (mebicarum) is an anxiolytic produced in Latvia and used in Eastern Europe. Mebicar has an effect on the structure of limbic-reticular activity, particularly on hypothalamus emotional zone, as well as on all 4 basic neuromediator systems – γ aminobutyric acid (GABA), choline, serotonin and adrenergic activity.[17] Mebicar decreases the brain noradrenaline level, exerts no effect on the dopaminergic systems, and increases the brain serotonin level.[18]

Fabomotizole   Fabomotizole[19] (brand name Afobazole) is an anxiolytic drug launched in Russia in the early 2000s. Its mechanism of action remains poorly defined, with GABAergic, NGF and BDNF release promoting, MT1 receptor antagonism, MT3 receptor antagonism, and sigma agonism all thought to have some involvement.[20][21][22][23][24] It has yet to find clinical use outside of Russia.

Selank   Selank is an anxiolytic peptide based drug developed by the Institute of Molecular Genetics of the Russian academy of sciences. Selank is a heptapeptide with the sequence Thr-Lys-Pro-Arg-Pro-Gly-Pro. It is a synthetic analog of a human tetrapeptide tuftsin. As such, it mimics many of its effects. It has been shown to modulate the expression of interleukin-6 (IL-6) and affect the balance of T helper cell cytokines. There is evidence that it may also modulate the expression of brain-derived neurotropic factor in rats.

Bromantane   Bromantane is a stimulant drug with anxiolytic properties developed in Russia during the late 1980s, which acts mainly by inhibiting the reuptake of both dopamine and serotonin in the brain, although it also has anticholinergic effects at very high doses. Study results suggest that the combination of psychostimulant and anxiolytic actions in the spectrum of psychotropic activity of bromantane is effective in treating asthenic disorders compared to placebo.

Emoxypine   Emoxypine is an antioxidant that is also an anxiolytic. Its chemical structure resembles that of pyridoxine, a type of vitamin B_6.

Azapirones   Azapirones are a class of 5-HT_1A receptor agonists. Currently approved azapirones include buspirone (Buspar) and tandospirone (Sediel).

Hydroxyzine   Hydroxyzine (Atarax) is an old antihistamine originally approved for clinical use by the FDA in 1956. It possesses anxiolytic properties in addition to its antihistamine properties and is also licensed for the treatment of anxiety and tension. It is also used for its sedative properties as a premed before anesthesia or to induce sedation after anesthesia.[25] It has been shown to be as effective as benzodiazepines in the treatment of generalized anxiety disorder, while producing fewer side-effects.[26]

Pregabalin   Pregabalin's therapeutic effect appears after 1 week of use and is similar in effectiveness to lorazepam, alprazolam, and venlafaxine, but pregabalin has demonstrated superiority by producing more consistent therapeutic effects for psychic and somatic anxiety symptoms. Long-term trials have shown continued effectiveness without the development of tolerance, and, in addition, unlike benzodiazepines, it does not disrupt sleep architecture and produces less severe cognitive and psychomotor impairment; it also has a low potential for abuse and dependence and may be preferred over the benzodiazepines for these reasons.[27][28]

Menthyl isovalerate   Menthyl isovalerate is a flavoring food additive which is marketed as a sedative and anxiolytic drug in Russia under the name *Validol*. Sublingual administration of *Validol* produces a sedative effect, and has moderate reflex and vascular dilative action caused by stimulation of sensory nerve receptors of the oral mucosa followed by the release of endorphins. *Validol* is typically administered *as needed* for symptom relief.[29][30][31]

Cannabidiol Cannabidiol (CBD) is a cannabinoid produced by *Cannabis sativa* and *Cannabis indica*, and in marginal quantities by *Cannabis ruderalis*. It is available in the United States in states where cannabis has been legalized for medical and general use. No lethal dose (or LD50) has been established from cannabidiol. In feral strains of cannabis, cannabidiol is produced in large quantities alongside the psychoactive cannabinoid tetrahydrocannabinol. Special strains of cannabis have been bred to yield high amounts of cannabidiol with significantly lowered synthesis of THC. Specific formulations for anxiety with a CBD to THC ratio of 18:1 are available in the US markets.

Tetrahydrocannabinol Tetrahydrocannabinol appears to be capable of both, having anxiolytic effect(s) and having anxiogenic effect(s).

Racetams Some racetam based drugs such as aniracetam can have an antianxiety effect.[32]

Herbal treatments

Certain natural substances are reputed to have anxiolytic properties, including the following:

- *Garcinia indica* (Kokum)[33]
- *Scutellaria lateriflora*[34]
- *Coriandrum sativum* (Coriander)[35]
- *Salvia elegans* (Pineapple Sage)[36]
- *Cannabidiol* (a cannabinoid found in marijuana)[37]

Supplements and over-the-counter pharmaceutical drugs

Picamilon is a prodrug formed by combining niacin with GABA that is able to cross the blood–brain barrier and is then hydrolyzed into GABA and niacin. It is theorized that the GABA released in this process activates GABA receptors, with potential to produce an anxiolytic response.[38][39] Picamilon is sold in the United States as a dietary supplement, while in Russia it is sold as a prescription drug.

Chlorpheniramine (Chlor-Trimeton)[40] and diphenhydramine (Benadryl) have hypnotic and sedative effects with mild anxiolytic-like properties (off-label use). These drugs are approved by the FDA for allergies, rhinitis, and urticaria.

Melatonin has anxiolytic properties, likely mediated by the benzodiazepine/GABAergic system.[41] It has been used experimentally as an effective premedicant for general anesthesia in surgical procedures.[42]

Inositol:[43] In a double-blind, controlled trial, *myo*-inositol (18 grams daily) was superior to fluvoxamine for decreasing the number of panic attacks and had fewer side-effects.[44]

Future drugs

Due to deficits with existing anxiolytics (either in terms of efficacy or side-effect profile), research into novel anxiolytics is active. Possible candidates for future drugs include:

- BNC210
- CL-218,872
- L-838,417
- SL-651,498
- S32212
- PH94B

Common drugs

Prescription-free drugs are often poor anxiolytics and often worsen the symptoms over time. However, they are often used for self-medication because of their wide availability (e.g. alcoholic beverages).

Alcohol See also: Short-term effects of alcohol

Ethanol is used as an anxiolytic, sometimes by self-medication. fMRI can measure the anxiolytic effects of alcohol in the human brain.[45] The British National Formulary states, "Alcohol is a poor hypnotic because its diuretic action interferes with sleep during the latter part of the night." Alcohol is also known to induce alcohol-related sleep disorders.[46]

Inhalants See also: Inhalant abuse § Patterns of nonmedical usage and Street children in Latin America § Drugs

The anxiolytic effects of solvents act as positive modulators of GABAA receptors (Bowen and colleagues 2006).[47]

1.3.3 See also

- ATC code N05#N05B Anxiolytics

1.3.4 References

[1] "antianxiety agent" at *Dorland's Medical Dictionary*

[2] Youngstedt, Shawn D; Kripke, Daniel F (2007). "Does bright light have an anxiolytic effect? - an open trial". *BMC Psychiatry* **7**: 62. doi:10.1186/1471-244X-7-62. PMC 2194679. PMID 17971237.

[3] Peggy E. Hayes; et al. (September–October 1987). "Beta-blockers in anxiety disorders". *Journal of Affective Disorders* **13** (2): 119–130.

[4] "anxiolytic (tranquilizer)". *Memidex (WordNet) Dictionary/Thesaurus*. Retrieved 2010-12-02.

[5] Zwanzger, P.; Deckert, J. (Mar 2007). "[Anxiety disorders. Causes, clinical picture and treatment]". *Nervenarzt* **78** (3): 349–59; quiz 360. doi:10.1007/s00115-006-2202-z. PMID 17279399.

[6] Shearer, SL. (Sep 2007). "Recent advances in the understanding and treatment of anxiety disorders". *Prim Care* **34** (3): 475–504, v–vi. doi:10.1016/j.pop.2007.05.002. PMID 17868756.

[7] Gould, RA; Otto, M; Pollack, M; Yap, L (1997). "Cognitive behavioral and pharmacological treatment of generalized anxiety disorder: A preliminary meta-analysis". *Behavior Therapy* **28** (2): 285–305. doi:10.1016/S0005-7894(97)80048-2.

[8] Pull, CB. (Jan 2007). "Combined pharmacotherapy and cognitive-behavioural therapy for anxiety disorders". *Curr Opin Psychiatry* **20** (1): 30–5. doi:10.1097/YCO.0b013e3280115e52. PMID 17143079.

[9] CMA & AMA Home medical guides 2012 & 2014, along with personal experiences and WebMD reviews

[10] Gelder, M, Mayou, R. and Geddes, J. 2005. Psychiatry. 3rd ed. New York: Oxford. pp236.

[11] Lader M, Tylee A, Donoghue J (2009). "Withdrawing benzodiazepines in primary care". *CNS Drugs* **23** (1): 19–34. doi:10.2165/0023210-200923010-00002. PMID 19062773.

[12] Montenegro, Mariana; Veiga, Heloisa; Deslandes, Andréa; Cagy, Maurício; McDowell, Kaleb; Pompeu, Fernando; Piedade, Roberto; Ribeiro, Pedro (2005). "Neuromodulatory effects of caffeine and bromazepam on visual event-related potential (P300): A comparative study". *Arquivos de Neuro-Psiquiatria* **63** (2b): 410–5. doi:10.1590/S0004-282X2005000300009. PMID 16059590.

[13] Barlow, David H. Durand, V. Mark (2009). "Chapter 7: Mood Disorders and Suicide". *Abnormal Psychology: An Integrative Approach* (Fifth ed.). Belmont, CA: Wadsworth Cengage Learning. p. 239. ISBN 0-495-09556-7. OCLC 192055408.

[14] John Vanin, James Helsley (19 June 2008). *Anxiety Disorders: A Pocket Guide For Primary Care*. Springer Science & Business Media. p. 189.

[15] Jefferson, J. W. (1974). Beta-adrenergic receptor blocking drugs in psychiatry. Archives of general psychiatry, 31(5), 681. doi:10.1001/archpsyc.1974.01760170071012 http://archpsyc.jamanetwork.com/article.aspx?articleid=491265

[16] Noyes Jr, R. (1982). Beta-blocking drugs and anxiety. Psychosomatics, 23(2), 155-170.

[17] "Adaptol. Summary of Product Characteristics" (PDF). Retrieved 24 July 2015.

[18] Val'Dman, AV; Zaikonnikova, IV; Kozlovskaia, MM; Zimakova, IE (1980). "Characteristics of the psychotropic spectrum of action of mebicar". *Biulleten' eksperimental'noi biologii i meditsiny* **89** (5): 568–70. PMID 6104993.

[19] "International Nonproprietary Names for Pharmaceutical Substances (INN)" (PDF). *WHO Drug Information* **26** (1): 63. 2012. Retrieved 21 March 2015.

[20] Neznamov, GG; Siuniakov, SA; Chumakov, DV; Bochkarev, VK; Seredenin, SB (2001). "Clinical study of the selective anxiolytic agent afobazol". *Eksperimental'naia i klinicheskaia farmakologiia* **64** (2): 15–9. PMID 11548440.

[21] Silkina, IV; Gan'shina, TC; Seredin, SB; Mirzoian, RS (2005). "Gabaergic mechanism of cerebrovascular and neuroprotective effects of afobazole and picamilon". *Eksperimental'naia i klinicheskaia farmakologiia* **68** (1): 20–4. PMID 15786959.

[22] Seredin, SB; Melkumian, DS; Val'dman, EA; Iarkova, MA; Seredina, TC; Voronin, MV; Lapitskaia, AS (2006). "Effects of afobazole on the BDNF content in brain structures of inbred mice with different phenotypes of emotional stress reaction". *Eksperimental'naia i klinicheskaia farmakologiia* **69** (3): 3–6. PMID 16878488.

[23] Antipova, TA; Sapozhnikova, DS; Bakhtina, LIu; Seredenin, SB (2009). "Selective anxiolytic afobazole increases the content of BDNF and NGF in cultured hippocampal HT-22 line neurons". *Eksperimental'naia i klinicheskaia farmakologiia* **72** (1): 12–4. PMID 19334503.

[24] Seredenin, SB; Antipova, TA; Voronin, MV; Kurchashova, SY; Kuimov, AN (2009). "Interaction of afobazole with sigma1-receptors". *Bulletin of experimental biology and medicine* **148** (1): 42–4. doi:10.1007/s10517-009-0624-x. PMID 19902093.

[25] medicine net. "hydroxyzine (Vistaril, Atarax)". medicinenet.com. Archived from the original on 13 May 2008. Retrieved 17 May 2008.

[26] Llorca PM, Spadone C, Sol O (November 2002). "Efficacy and safety of hydroxyzine in the treatment of generalized anxiety disorder: a 3-month double-blind study". *J Clin Psychiatry* **63** (11): 1020–7. doi:10.4088/JCP.v63n1112. PMID 12444816.

[27] Bandelow, B.; Wedekind, D.; Leon, T. (Jul 2007). "Pregabalin for the treatment of generalized anxiety disorder: a novel pharmacologic intervention". *Expert Rev Neurother* **7** (7): 769–81. doi:10.1586/14737175.7.7.769. PMID 17610384.

[28] Owen, RT. (Sep 2007). "Pregabalin: its efficacy, safety and tolerability profile in generalized anxiety". *Drugs Today (Barc)* **43** (9): 601–10. doi:10.1358/dot.2007.43.9.1133188. PMID 17940637.

[29] The Great Soviet Encyclopedia http://encyclopedia2.thefreedictionary.com/Validol[]

[30] Farmak Product Information - Validol http://farmak.ua/assets_images/drugs/instruction/en/25/Validol_Product_Information.pdf[]

[31] Itop Doctor http://doctor.itop.net/DirectoryItem.aspx?DirId=1&ItemId=268[]

[32] Malykh AG; Sadaie MR (Feb 2010). "Piracetam and piracetam-like drugs: from basic science to novel clinical applications to CNS disorders.". *Drugs.* **70** (3): 287–312. doi:10.2165/11319230-000000000-00000. PMID 20166767.

[33] Patel, Manish; Antala, Bhavesh; Barua, Chandana; Lahkar, Mangala (2013). "Anxiolytic activity of aqueous extract of *Garcinia indica* in mice". *International Journal of Green Pharmacy* **7** (4): 332–35. doi:10.4103/0973-8258.122089.

[34] Wolfson, P; Hoffmann, DL (2003). "An investigation into the efficacy of Scutellaria lateriflora in healthy volunteers". *Alternative therapies in health and medicine* **9** (2): 74–8. PMID 12652886.

[35] Emamghoreishi M, Khasaki M, Aazam MF (2005). "Coriandrum sativum: evaluation of its anxiolytic effect in the elevated plus-maze". *Journal of Ethnopharmacology* **96** (3): 365–370. doi:10.1016/j.jep.2004.06.022. PMID 15619553.

[36] Herrera-Ruiz, Maribel; García-Beltrán, Yolanda; Mora, Sergio; Díaz-Véliz, Gabriela; Viana, Glauce S.B.; Tortoriello, Jaime; Ramírez, Guillermo (2006). "Antidepressant and anxiolytic effects of hydroalcoholic extract from Salvia elegans". *Journal of Ethnopharmacology* **107** (1): 53–8. doi:10.1016/j.jep.2006.02.003. PMID 16530995.

[37] Zuardi, A.W.; Crippa, J.A.S.; Hallak, J.E.C.; Moreira, F.A.; Guimarães, F.S. (2006). "Cannabidiol, a Cannabis sativa constituent, as an antipsychotic drug". *Brazilian Journal of Medical and Biological Research* **39** (4): 421–9. doi:10.1590/S0100-879X2006000400001. PMID 16612464.

[38] Shephard RA (June 1987). "Behavioral effects of GABA agonists in relation to anxiety and benzodiazepine action". *Life Sci.* **40** (25): 2429–36. doi:10.1016/0024-3205(87)90758-2. PMID 2884549.

[39] Foster AC, Kemp JA (February 2006). "Glutamate- and GABA-based CNS therapeutics". *Curr Opin Pharmacol* **6** (1): 7–17. doi:10.1016/j.coph.2005.11.005. PMID 16377242.

[40] Miyata, Shigeo; Hirano, Shoko; Ohsawa, Masahiro; Kamei, Junzo (2009). "Chlorpheniramine exerts anxiolytic-like effects and activates prefrontal 5-HT systems in mice". *Psychopharmacology* **213** (2–3): 441–52. doi:10.1007/s00213-009-1695-0. PMID 19823805.

[41] Pierrefiche, G; Zerbib, R; Laborit, H (1993). "Anxiolytic activity of melatonin in mice: Involvement of benzodiazepine receptors". *Research communications in chemical pathology and pharmacology* **82** (2): 131–42. PMID 7905658.

[42] Naguib, Mohamed; Gottumukkala, Vijaya; Goldstein, Peter A. (2007). "Melatonin and anesthesia: A clinical perspective". *Journal of Pineal Research* **42** (1): 12–21. doi:10.1111/j.1600-079X.2006.00384.x. PMID 17198534.

[43] Fux M, Levine J, Aviv A, Belmaker RH (1996). "Inositol treatment of obsessive-compulsive disorder". *American Journal of Psychiatry* **153** (9): 1219–1221. PMID 8780431.

[44] Palatnik A, Frolov K, Fux M, Benjamin J (2001). "Double-blind, controlled, crossover trial of inositol versus fluvoxamine for the treatment of panic disorder". *Journal of Clinical Psychopharmacology* **21** (3): 335–339. doi:10.1097/00004714-200106000-00014. PMID 11386498.

[45] Gilman, J. M.; Ramchandani, V. A.; Davis, M. B.; Bjork, J. M.; Hommer, D. W. (2008). "Why We Like to Drink: A Functional Magnetic Resonance Imaging Study of the Rewarding and Anxiolytic Effects of Alcohol". *Journal of Neuroscience* **28** (18): 4583–91. doi:10.1523/JNEUROSCI.0086-08.2008. PMC 2730732. PMID 18448634.

[46] http://pubs.niaaa.nih.gov/publications/aa41.htm[]

[47] Howard, Matthew O.; Bowen, Scott E.; Garland, Eric L.; Perron, Brian E.; Vaughn, Michael G. (2011). "Inhalant use and inhalant use disorders in the United States". *Addiction science & clinical practice* **6** (1): 18–31. PMC 3188822. PMID 22003419.

Chapter 2

Related Articles & Precautions

2.1 Benzodiazepine overdose

Benzodiazepine overdose describes the ingestion of one of the drugs in the benzodiazepine class in quantities greater than are recommended or generally practiced. Death as a result of taking an excessive dose of benzodiazepines alone is uncommon (versus combined drug intoxication) but does occasionally happen.[1] Deaths after hospital admission are considered to be low.[2] However, combinations of high doses of benzodiazepines with alcohol, barbiturates, opioids or tricyclic antidepressants are particularly dangerous, and may lead to severe complications such as coma or death. The most common symptoms of overdose include central nervous system (CNS) depression and intoxication with impaired balance, ataxia, and slurred speech. Severe symptoms include coma and respiratory depression. Supportive care is the mainstay of treatment of benzodiazepine overdose. There is an antidote, flumazenil, but its use is controversial.[3]

As benzodiazepines are one of the most highly prescribed classes of drugs[4] they are commonly used in self-poisoning by drug overdose.[5][6] The various benzodiazepines differ in their toxicity since they produce varying levels of sedation in overdose. A 1993 British study of deaths during the 1980s found flurazepam and temazepam more frequently involved in drug-related deaths, causing more deaths per million prescriptions than other benzodiazepines. Flurazepam, now rarely prescribed in the United Kingdom and Australia, had the highest fatal toxicity index of any benzodiazepine (15.0), followed by temazepam (11.9), versus benzodiazepines overall (5.9), taken with or without alcohol.[7] An Australian (1995) study found oxazepam less toxic and less sedative, and temazepam more toxic and more sedative, than most benzodiazepines in overdose.[8] An Australian study (2004) of overdose admissions between 1987 and 2002 found alprazolam, which happens to be the most prescribed benzodiazepine in the U.S. by a large margin, to be more toxic than diazepam and other benzodiazepines. They also cited a review of the Annual Reports of the American Association of Poison Control Centers National Data Collection System, which showed alprazolam was involved in 34 fatal deliberate self-poisonings over 10 years (1992–2001), compared with 30 fatal deliberate self-poisonings involving diazepam.[9] In a New Zealand study (2003) of 200 deaths, Zopiclone, a benzodiazepine receptor agonist, had similar overdose potential as benzodiazepines.[10]

2.1.1 Signs and symptoms

Following an acute overdose of a benzodiazepine the onset of symptoms is typically rapid with most developing symptoms within 4 hours.[11] Patients initially present with mild to moderate impairment of central nervous system function. Initial signs and symptoms include intoxication, somnolence, diplopia, impaired balance, impaired motor function, anterograde amnesia, ataxia, and slurred speech. Most patients with pure benzodiazepine overdose will usually only exhibit these mild CNS symptoms.[11][12] Paradoxical reactions such as anxiety, delirium, combativeness, hallucinations, and aggression can also occur following benzodiazepine overdose.[13] Gastrointestinal symptoms such as nausea and vomiting have also been occasionally reported.[12]

Cases of severe overdose have been reported and symptoms displayed may include prolonged deep coma or deep cyclic coma, apnea, respiratory depression, hypoxemia, hypothermia, hypotension, bradycardia, cardiac arrest, and pulmonary aspiration, with the possibility of death.[11][14][15][16][17][18] Severe consequences are rare following overdose of benzodiazepines alone but the severity of overdose is increased significantly if benzodiazepines are taken in overdose in combination with other medications.[18] Significant toxicity may result following recreation drug misuse in conjunction with other CNS depressants such as opioids or ethanol.[19][20][21][22] The duration of symptoms following overdose is usually between 12 and 36 hours in the majority of cases.[12] The majority of drug-related deaths involve misuse of heroin or other opioids in combination with benzodiazepines or other CNS depressant drugs. In most cases of fatal overdose it is likely that lack of opioid tolerance combined with the depressant effects of benzodiazepines in the cause of death.[23]

The symptoms of an overdose such as sleepiness, agitation and ataxia occur much more frequently and severely in children. Hypotonia may also occur in severe cases.[24]

2.1.2 Toxicity

Benzodiazepines have a wide therapeutic index and taken alone in overdose rarely cause severe complications or fatalities.[12][25] More often than not, a patient who inadvertently takes more than the prescribed dose will simply feel drowsy and fall asleep for a few hours. Of course, patients who are suicidal can easily take dosages that will become lethal once absorbed into the body. Benzodiazepines taken in overdose in combination with alcohol, barbiturates, opioids, tricyclic antidepressants, or sedating antipsychotics, anticonvulsants, or antihistamines are particularly dangerous.[26] In the case of alcohol and barbiturates, not only do they have an additive effect but they also increase the binding affinity of benzodiazepines to the benzodiazepine binding site, which results in a very significant potentiation of the CNS and respiratory depressant effects.[27][28][29][30][31] In addition, the elderly and those with chronic illnesses are much more vulnerable to lethal overdose with benzodiazepines. Fatal overdoses can occur at relatively low doses in these individuals.[12][32][33][34]

2.1.3 Pathophysiology

Benzodiazepines bind to a specific benzodiazepine receptor, thereby enhancing the effect of the neurotransmitter gamma-aminobutyric acid (GABA) and causing CNS depression. In overdose situations this pharmacological effect is extended leading to a more severe CNS depression and potentially coma [12] or cardiac arrest.[35] Benzodiazepine-overdose-related coma may be characterised by an alpha pattern with the central somatosensory conduction time (CCT) after median nerve stimulation being prolonged and the N20 to be dispersed. Brain-stem auditory evoked potentials demonstrate delayed interpeak latencies (IPLs) I-III, III-V and I-V. Toxic overdoses of benzodiazepines therefore cause prolonged CCT and IPLs.[36][37][38]

2.1.4 Diagnosis

The diagnosis of benzodiazepine overdose may be difficult, but is usually made based on the clinical presentation of the patient along with a history of overdose.[12][39] Obtaining a laboratory test for benzodiazepine blood concentrations can be useful in patients presenting with CNS depression or coma of unknown origin. Techniques available to measure blood concentrations include thin layer chromatography, gas liquid chromatography with or without a mass spectrometer, and radioimmunoassay.[12] Blood benzodiazepine concentrations, however, do not appear to be related to any toxicological effect or predictive of clinical outcome. Blood concentrations are, therefore, used mainly to confirm the diagnosis rather than being useful for the clinical management of the patient.[12][40]

2.1.5 Treatment

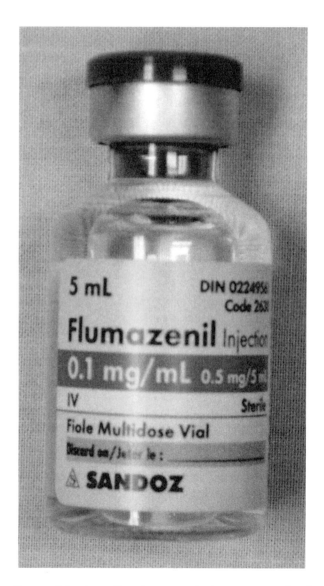

Flumazenil is a benzodiazepine antagonist that can reverse the effects of benzodiazepines, although its use following benzodiazepine overdose is controversial.

Medical observation and supportive care are the mainstay of treatment of benzodiazepine overdose.[41] Although benzodiazepines are absorbed by activated charcoal,[42] gastric decontamination with activated charcoal is not beneficial in pure benzodiazepine overdose as the risk of adverse effects would outweigh any potential benefit from the procedure. It is recommended only if benzodiazepines have been taken in combination with other drugs that may benefit from decontamination.[43] Gastric lavage (stomach pumping) or whole bowel irrigation are also not recommended.[43] Enhancing elimination of the drug with hemodialysis, hemoperfusion, or forced diuresis is unlikely to be beneficial as these procedures have little effect on the clearance of benzodiazepines due to their large volume of distribution and lipid solubility.[43]

Supportive measures

Supportive measures include observation of vital signs, especially Glasgow Coma Scale and airway patency. IV access with fluid administration and maintenance of the airway with intubation and artificial ventilation may be required if respiratory depression or pulmonary aspiration occurs.[43] Supportive measures should be put in place prior to administration of any benzodiazepine antagonist in order to protect the patient from both the withdrawal effects and possible complications arising from the benzodiazepine. A determination of possible deliberate overdose should be considered with appropriate scrutiny, and precautions taken to prevent any attempt by the patient to commit further bodily harm.[8][44] Hypotension is corrected with fluid replacement, although catecholamines such as norepinephrine or dopamine may be required to increase blood pressure.[12] Bradycardia is treated with atropine or an infusion of norepinephrine to increase coronary blood flow and heart rate.[12]

Flumazenil

Flumazenil (Anexate) is a competitive benzodiazepine receptor antagonist that can be used as an antidote for benzodiazepine overdose. Its use, however, is controversial as it has numerous contraindications.[3][45] It is contraindicated in patients who are on long-term benzodiazepines, those who have ingested a substance that lowers the seizure threshold, or in patients who have tachycardia, widened QRS complex on ECG, anticholinergic signs, or a history of seizures.[46] Due to these contraindications and the possibility of it causing severe adverse effects including seizures, adverse cardiac effects, and death,[47][48] in the majority of cases there is no indication for the use of flumazenil in the management of benzodiazepine overdose as the risks in general outweigh any potential benefit of administration.[3][43] It also has no role in the management of unknown overdoses.[5][45] In addition, if full airway protection has been achieved, a good outcome is expected, and therefore flumazenil administration is unlikely to be required.[49]

Flumazenil is very effective at reversing the CNS depression associated with benzodiazepines but is less effective at reversing respiratory depression.[45] One study found that only 10% of the patient population presenting with a benzodiazepine overdose are suitable candidates for flumazenil.[45] In this select population who are naive to and overdose solely on a benzodiazepine, it can be considered.[50] Due to its short half life, the duration of action of flumazenil is usually less than 1 hour, and multiple doses may be needed.[45] When flumazenil is indicated the risks can be reduced or avoided by slow dose titration of flumazenil.[44] Due to risks and its many contraindications, flumazenil should be administered only after discussion with a medical toxicologist.[50][51]

2.1.6 Epidemiology

In a Swedish (2003) study benzodiazepines were implicated in 39% of suicides by drug poisoning in the elderly 1992-1996. Nitrazepam and flunitrazepam accounted for 90% of benzodiazepine implicated suicides. In cases where benzodiazepines contributed to death, but were not the sole cause, drowning, typically in the bath, was a common method used. Benzodiazepines were the predominant drug class in suicides in this review of Swedish death certificates. In 72% of the cases, benzodiazepines were the only drug consumed. Thus, many of deaths associated with benzodiazepine overdoses may not be a direct result of the toxic effects but either due to being combined with other drugs or used as a tool to complete suicide using a different method, e.g. drowning.[52]

In a Swedish retrospective study of deaths of 1987, in 159 of 1587 autopsy cases benzodiazepines were found. In 44 of these cases the cause of death was natural causes or unclear. The remaining 115 deaths were due to accidents (N = 16), suicide (N = 60), drug addiction (N = 29) or alcoholism (N = 10). In a comparison of suicides and natural deaths, the concentrations both of flunitrazepam and nitrazepam (sleeping medications) were significantly higher among the suicides. In four cases benzodiazepines were the sole cause of death.[53]

In Australia, a study of 16 deaths associated with toxic concentrations of benzodiazepines during the period of 5 years leading up to July 1994 found preexisting natural disease as a feature of 11 cases; 14 cases were suicides. Cases where other drugs, including ethanol, had contributed to the death were excluded. In the remaining five cases, death was caused solely by benzodiazepines. Nitrazepam and temazepam were the most prevalent drugs detected, followed by oxazepam and flunitrazepam.[54] A review of self poisonings of 12 months 1976 - 1977 in Auckland, New Zealand, found benzodiazepines implicated in 40% of the cases.[55] A 1993 British study found flurazepam and temazepam to have the highest number of deaths per million prescriptions among medications commonly prescribed in the 1980s. Flurazepam, now rarely prescribed in the United Kingdom and Australia, had the highest fatal toxicity index of any benzodiazepine (15.0) followed by Temazepam (11.9), versus 5.9 for benzodiazepines overall, taken with or without alcohol.[7]

2.1.7 References

[1] Dart, Richard C. (1 December 2003). *Medical Toxicology* (3rd ed.). USA: Lippincott Williams & Wilkins. p. 811. ISBN 978-0-7817-2845-4.

[2] Höjer J, Baehrendtz S, Gustafsson L (August 1989). "Benzodiazepine poisoning: experience of 702 admissions to an intensive care unit during a 14-year period". *J. Intern. Med.* **226** (2): 117–22. doi:10.1111/j.1365-2796.1989.tb01365.x. PMID 2769176.

[3] Seger DL (2004). "Flumazenil--treatment or toxin". *J. Toxicol. Clin. Toxicol.* **42** (2): 209–16. doi:10.1081/CLT-120030946. PMID 15214628.

[4] Taylor S, McCracken CF, Wilson KC, Copeland JR (November 1998). "Extent and appropriateness of benzodiazepine use. Results from an elderly urban community". *Br J Psychiatry* **173** (5): 433–8. doi:10.1192/bjp.173.5.433. PMID 9926062.

[5] Ngo AS, Anthony CR, Samuel M, Wong E, Ponampalam R (July 2007). "Should a benzodiazepine antagonist be used in unconscious patients presenting to the emergency department?". *Resuscitation* **74** (1): 27–37. doi:10.1016/j.resuscitation.2006.11.010. PMID 17306436.

[6] Jonasson B, Jonasson U, Saldeen T (January 2000). "Among fatal poisonings dextropropoxyphene predominates in younger people, antidepressants in the middle aged and sedatives in the elderly". *J. Forensic Sci.* **45** (1): 7–10. PMID 10641912.

[7] Serfaty M, Masterton G (January 1994). "Fatal poisonings attributed to benzodiazepines in Britain during the 1980s". *British Journal of Psychiatry* **163** (3): 386–93. doi:10.1192/bjp.163.3.386. PMID 8104653.

[8] Buckley NA, Dawson AH, Whyte IM, O'Connell DL (28 January 1995). "Relative toxicity of benzodiazepines in overdose". *BMJ* **310** (6974): 219–21. doi:10.1136/bmj.310.6974.219. PMC 2548618. PMID 7866122.

[9] Isbister GK, O'Regan L, Sibbritt D, Whyte IM (July 2004). "Alprazolam is relatively more toxic than other benzodiazepines in overdose". *Br J Clin Pharmacol* **58** (1): 88–95. doi:10.1111/j.1365-2125.2004.02089.x. PMC 1884537. PMID 15206998.

[10] Reith DM, Fountain J, McDowell R, Tilyard M (2003). "Comparison of the fatal toxicity index of zopiclone with benzodiazepines". *J. Toxicol. Clin. Toxicol.* **41** (7): 975–80. doi:10.1081/CLT-120026520. PMID 14705844.

[11] Wiley CC, Wiley JF (1998). "Pediatric benzodiazepine ingestion resulting in hospitalization". *J. Toxicol. Clin. Toxicol.* **36** (3): 227–31. doi:10.3109/15563659809028944. PMID 9656979.

[12] Gaudreault P, Guay J, Thivierge RL, Verdy I (1991). "Benzodiazepine poisoning. Clinical and pharmacological considerations and treatment". *Drug Saf* **6** (4): 247–65. doi:10.2165/00002018-199106040-00003. PMID 1888441.

[13] Garnier R, Medernach C, Harbach S, Fournier E (April 1984). "[Agitation and hallucinations during acute lorazepam poisoning in children. Apropos of 65 personal cases]". *Ann Pediatr (Paris)* (in French) **31** (4): 286–9. PMID 6742700.

[14] Berger R, Green G, Melnick A (September 1975). "Cardiac arrest caused by oral diazepam intoxication". *Clin Pediatr (Phila)* **14** (9): 842–4. doi:10.1177/000992287501400910. PMID 1157438.

[15] Welch TR, Rumack BH, Hammond K (1977). "Clonazepam overdose resulting in cyclic coma". *Clin. Toxicol.* **10** (4): 433–6. doi:10.3109/15563657709046280. PMID 862377.

[16] Höjer J, Baehrendtz S, Gustafsson L (August 1989). "Benzodiazepine poisoning: experience of 702 admissions to an intensive care unit during a 14-year period". *J. Intern. Med.* **226** (2): 117–22. doi:10.1111/j.1365-2796.1989.tb01365.x. PMID 2769176.

[17] Busto U, Kaplan HL, Sellers EM (February 1980). "Benzodiazepine-associated emergencies in Toronto". *Am J Psychiatry* **137** (2): 224–7. PMID 6101526.

[18] Greenblatt DJ, Allen MD, Noel BJ, Shader RI (April 1977). "Acute overdosage with benzodiazepine derivatives". *Clin. Pharmacol. Ther.* **21** (4): 497–514. PMID 14802.

[19] Lai SH; Yao YJ; Lo DS (October 2006). "A survey of buprenorphine related deaths in Singapore". *Forensic Sci Int* **162** (1–3): 80–6. doi:10.1016/j.forsciint.2006.03.037. PMID 16879940.

[20] Koski A, Ojanperä I, Vuori E (May 2003). "Interaction of alcohol and drugs in fatal poisonings". *Hum Exp Toxicol* **22** (5): 281–7. doi:10.1191/0960327103ht324oa. PMID 12774892.

[21] Wishart, David (2006). "Triazolam". *DrugBank*. Retrieved 2006-03-23.

[22] Hung DZ, Tsai WJ, Deng JF (July 1992). "Anterograde amnesia in triazolam overdose despite flumazenil treatment: a case report". *Hum Exp Toxicol* **11** (4): 289–90. doi:10.1177/096032719201100410. PMID 1354979.

[23] National Treatment Agency for Substance Misuse (2007). "Drug misuse and dependence - UK guidelines on clinical management" (PDF). United Kingdom: Department of Health.

[24] Pulce C, Mollon P, Pham E, Frantz P, Descotes J (April 1992). "Acute poisonings with ethyle loflazepate, flunitrazepam, prazepam and triazolam in children". *Vet Hum Toxicol* **34** (2): 141–3. PMID 1354907.

[25] Wolf BC, Lavezzi WA, Sullivan LM, Middleberg RA, Flannagan LM (2005). "Alprazolam-related deaths in Palm Beach County". *Am J Forensic Med Pathol* **26** (1): 24–7. doi:10.1097/01.paf.0000153994.95642.c1. PMID 15725773.

[26] Charlson F, Degenhardt L, McLaren J, Hall W, Lynskey M (February 2009). "A systematic review of research examining benzodiazepine-related mortality". *Pharmacoepidemiol Drug Saf* **18** (2): 93–103. doi:10.1002/pds.1694. PMID 19125401.

[27] Dietze P, Jolley D, Fry C, Bammer G (May 2005). "Transient changes in behaviour lead to heroin overdose: results from a case-crossover study of non-fatal overdose". *Addiction* **100** (5): 636–42. doi:10.1111/j.1360-0443.2005.01051.x. PMID 15847621.

[28] Hammersley R; Cassidy MT; Oliver J (July 1995). "Drugs associated with drug-related deaths in Edinburgh and Glasgow, November 1990 to October 1992". *Addiction* **90** (7): 959–65. doi:10.1046/j.1360-0443.1995.9079598.x. PMID 7663317.

[29] Ticku MK, Burch TP, Davis WC (1983). "The interactions of ethanol with the benzodiazepine-GABA receptor-ionophore complex". *Pharmacol. Biochem. Behav.* 18 Suppl 1: 15–8. doi:10.1016/0091-3057(83)90140-5. PMID 6138771.

[30] Kudo K, Imamura T, Jitsufuchi N, Zhang XX, Tokunaga H, Nagata T (April 1997). "Death attributed to the toxic interaction of triazolam, amitriptyline and other psychotropic drugs". *Forensic Sci. Int.* **86** (1–2): 35–41. doi:10.1016/S0379-0738(97)02110-5. PMID 9153780.

[31] Rogers, Wo; Hall, Ma; Brissie, Rm; Robinson, Ca (Jan 1997). "Detection of alprazolam in three cases of methadone/benzodiazepine overdose". *Journal of forensic sciences* **42** (1): 155–6. ISSN 0022-1198. PMID 8988593.

[32] Sunter JP, Bal TS, Cowan WK (September 1988). "Three cases of fatal triazolam poisoning". *BMJ* **297** (6650): 719. doi:10.1136/bmj.297.6650.719. PMC 1834083. PMID 3147739.

[33] Brødsgaard I; Hansen AC; Vesterby A (June 1995). "Two cases of lethal nitrazepam poisoning". *Am J Forensic Med Pathol* **16** (2): 151–3. doi:10.1097/00000433-199506000-00015. PMID 7572872.

[34] Reidenberg MM, Levy M, Warner H, Coutinho CB, Schwartz MA, Yu G, Cheripko J (April 1978). "Relationship between diazepam dose, plasma level, age, and central nervous system depression". *Clin. Pharmacol. Ther.* **23** (4): 371–4. PMID 630787.

[35] Berger, R,; Green G; Melnick A. (1975). "Cardiac Arrest Caused by Oral Diazepam Intoxication". *Clinical Pediatrics* **14** (9): 842–844. doi:10.1177/000992287501400910. PMID 1157438.

[36] Rumpl E; Prugger M; Battista HJ; Badry F; Gerstenbrand F; Dienstl F (December 1988). "Short latency somatosensory evoked potentials and brain-stem auditory evoked potentials in coma due to CNS depressant drug poisoning. Preliminary observations". *Electroencephalography and clinical neurophysiology* **70** (6): 482–9. doi:10.1016/0013-4694(88)90146-0. PMID 2461282.

[37] Pasinato, E; Franciosi, A; De, Vanna, M (Apr 1983). ""Alpha pattern coma" after poisoning with flunitrazepam and bromazepam. Case description". *Minerva psichiatrica* **24** (2): 69–74. ISSN 0374-9320. PMID 6140613.

[38] Carroll WM, Mastiglia FL (December 1977). "Alpha and beta coma in drug intoxication" (PDF). *Br Med J* **2** (6101): 1518–9. doi:10.1136/bmj.2.6101.1518-a. PMC 1632784. PMID 589310.

[39] Perry HE, Shannon MW (June 1996). "Diagnosis and management of opioid- and benzodiazepine-induced comatose overdose in children". *Current Opinion in Pediatrics* **8** (3): 243–7. doi:10.1097/00008480-199606000-00010. PMID 8814402.

[40] Jatlow P, Dobular K, Bailey D (October 1979). "Serum diazepam concentrations in overdose. Their significance". *Am. J. Clin. Pathol.* **72** (4): 571–7. PMID 40432.

[41] Welch TR, Rumack BH, Hammond K (1977). "Clonazepam overdose resulting in cyclic coma". *Clin. Toxicol.* **10** (4): 433–6. doi:10.3109/15563657709046280. PMID 862377.

[42] el-Khordagui LK, Saleh AM, KhalIl SA (1987). "Adsorption of benzodiazepines on charcoal and its correlation with in vitro and in vivo data". *Pharm Acta Helv* **62** (1): 28–32. PMID 2882522.

[43] Whyte, IM (2004). "Benzodiazepines". *Medical toxicology*. Philadelphia: Williams & Wilkins. pp. 811–22. ISBN 0-7817-2845-2.

[44] Weinbroum AA, Flaishon R, Sorkine P, Szold O, Rudick V (September 1997). "A risk-benefit assessment of flumazenil in the management of benzodiazepine overdose". *Drug Saf* **17** (3): 181–96. doi:10.2165/00002018-199717030-00004. PMID 9306053.

[45] Nelson, LH; Flomenbaum N; Goldfrank LR; Hoffman RL; Howland MD; Neal AL (2006). "Antidotes in depth: Flumazenil". *Goldfrank's toxicologic emergencies* (8th ed.). New York: McGraw-Hill. pp. 1112–7. ISBN 0-07-147914-7.

[46] Spivey WH (1992). "Flumazenil and seizures: analysis of 43 cases". *Clin Ther* **14** (2): 292–305. PMID 1611650.

[47] Marchant B, Wray R, Leach A, Nama M (September 1989). "Flumazenil causing convulsions and ventricular tachycardia". *BMJ* **299** (6703): 860. doi:10.1136/bmj.299.6703.860-b. PMC 1837717. PMID 2510872.

[48] Burr W, Sandham P, Judd A (June 1989). "Death after flumazepil". *BMJ* **298** (6689): 1713. doi:10.1136/bmj.298.6689.1713-a. PMC 1836759. PMID 2569340.

[49] Hoffman RS, Goldfrank LR (August 1995). "The poisoned patient with altered consciousness. Controversies in the use of a 'coma cocktail'". *JAMA* **274** (7): 562–9. doi:10.1001/jama.274.7.562. PMID 7629986.

[50] Nelson LH, Flomenbaum N, Goldfrank LR, Hoffman RL, Howland MD, Neal AL (2006). "Sedative-hypnotic agents". *Goldfrank's toxicologic emergencies* (8th ed.). New York: McGraw-Hill. pp. 929–51. ISBN 0-07-147914-7.

[51] Thomson JS, Donald C, Lewin K (February 2006). "Use of Flumazenil in benzodiazepine overdose". *Emerg Med J* **23** (2): 162. PMC 2564056. PMID 16439763.

[52] Carlsten, A; Waern M; Holmgren P; Allebeck P (2003). "The role of benzodiazepines in elderly suicides". *Scand J Public Health* **31** (3): 224–8. doi:10.1080/14034940210167966. PMID 12850977.

[53] Ericsson HR; Holmgren P; Jakobsson SW; Lafolie P; De Rees B (November 10, 1993). "Benzodiazepine findings in autopsy material. A study shows interacting factors in fatal cases". *Läkartidningen* **90** (45): 3954–7. PMID 8231567.

[54] Drummer OH; Ranson DL (December 1996). "Sudden death and benzodiazepines". *Am J Forensic Med Pathol* **17** (4): 336–42. doi:10.1097/00000433-199612000-00012. PMID 8947361.

[55] Large RG (September 1978). "Self-poisoning in Auckland reconsidered". *N. Z. Med. J.* **88** (620): 240–3. PMID 31581.

2.2 Benzodiazepine dependence

Benzodiazepine dependence or **benzodiazepine addiction** is when one has developed one or more of either tolerance, withdrawal symptoms, drug seeking behaviors, such as continued use despite harmful effects, and maladaptive pattern of substance use, according to the DSM-IV. In the case of benzodiazepine dependence, however, the continued use seems to be associated with the avoidance of unpleasant withdrawal reaction rather than from the pleasurable effects of the drug.[1] Benzodiazepine dependence develops with long-term use, even at low therapeutic doses,[2] without the described dependence behavior.[3][4]

Addiction, or what is sometimes referred to as psychological dependence, includes people misusing or craving the drug not to relieve withdrawal symptoms, but to experience its euphoric or intoxicating effects. It is important to distinguish between addiction and drug abuse of benzodiazepines and normal physical dependence on benzodiazepines. The increased GABAA inhibition caused by benzodiazepines is counteracted by the body's development of tolerance to the drug's effects; the development of tolerance occurs as a result of neuroadaptations, which result in decreased GABA inhibition and increased excitability of the glutamate system; these adaptations occur as a result of the body trying to overcome the central nervous system depressant effects of the drug to restore homeostasis. When benzodiazepines are stopped, these neuroadaptations are "unmasked" leading to hyper-excitability of the nervous system and the appearance of withdrawal symptoms.[5]

Therapeutic dose dependence is the largest category of people dependent on benzodiazepines. These individuals typically do not escalate their doses to high levels or abuse their medication. Smaller groups include patients escalating their dosage to higher levels and drug misusers as well. It is unclear exactly how many people illicitly abuse benzodiazepines. Tolerance develops within days or weeks to the anticonvulsant, hypnotic muscle relaxant and after 4 months there is little evidence that benzodiazepines retain their anxiolytic properties. Some authors, however, disagree and feel that benzodiazepines retain their anxiolytic properties.[6] Long-term benzodiazepine treatment may remain necessary in certain clinical conditions.[7]

Dependence and misuse of benzodiazepines have been of concern since 2002. Based on findings in the US from the Treatment Episode Data Set (TEDS), an annual compilation of patient characteristics in substance abuse treatment facilities in the United States, admissions due to "primary tranquilizer" (including, but not limited to, benzodiazepine-type) drug use increased 79% from 1992 to 2002. Thus, the DAWN and TEDS data sets demonstrate clearly that the misuse of these sedative/hypnotics is on the rise, and cause for concern.[8]

Numbers of benzodiazepine prescriptions have been declining, due primarily to concerns of dependence. In the short term, benzodiazepines can be effective drugs for acute anxiety or insomnia. With longer-term use, other therapies, both pharmacological and psychotherapeutic, become more effective. This is in part due to the greater effectiveness over time of other forms of therapy, and also due to the eventual development of pharmacological benzodiazepine tolerance.[9][10]

2.2.1 Definition

Benzodiazepine dependence is the condition resulting from repeated use of benzodiazepine drugs. It can include both a physical dependence as well as a psychological dependence and is typified by a withdrawal syndrome upon a fall in blood plasma levels of benzodiazepines, e.g., during dose reduction or abrupt withdrawal.[11]

2.2.2 Signs and symptoms

See also: Benzodiazepine withdrawal syndrome § Signs and symptoms

The signs and symptoms of benzodiazepine dependence include feeling unable to cope without the drug, unsuccessful attempts to cut down or stop benzodiazepine use, tolerance to the effects of benzodiazepines, and withdrawal symptoms when not taking the drug. Some withdrawal symptoms that may appear include anxiety, depressed mood, depersonalisation, derealisation, sleep disturbance, hypersensitivity to touch and pain, tremor, shakiness, muscular aches, pains, twitches, and headache.[12] Benzodiazepine dependence and withdrawal have been associated with suicide and self-harming behaviors, especially in young people. The Department of Health substance misuse guidelines recommend monitoring for mood disorder in those dependent on or withdrawing from benzodiazepines.[13]

Benzodiazepine dependence is a frequent complication for those prescribed for or using for longer than four weeks, with physical dependence and withdrawal symptoms being the most common problem, but also occasionally drug-seeking behavior. Withdrawal symptoms include anxiety, perceptual disturbances, distortion of all the senses, dysphoria, and, in rare cases, psychosis and epileptic seizures.[14]

2.2.3 Cause

Tolerance occurs to the muscle-relaxant, anticonvulsant, and sleep-inducing effects of benzodiazepines, and upon cessation a benzodiazepine withdrawal syndrome occurs. This can lead to benzodiazepines being taken for longer than originally intended, as people continue to take the drugs over a long period of time to suppress withdrawal symptoms. Some people abuse benzodiazepines at very high doses and devote a lot of time to doing so, satisfying the diagnostic criteria in DSM IV for substance abuse and dependence. Another group of people include those on low to moderate therapeutic doses of benzodiazepines who do not abuse their benzodiazepines but develop a tolerance and benzodiazepine dependence.[5] A considerable number of individuals using benzodiazepines for insomnia escalate their dosage, sometimes above therapeutically-prescribed dose levels. Tolerance to the anxiolytic effect of benzodiazepines has been clearly demonstrated in rats. In humans, there is little evidence that benzodiazepines retain their anti-anxiety effects beyond four months of continuous treatment; there is evidence that suggests that long-term use of benzodiazepines may actually worsen anxiety, which in turn may lead to dosage escalation, with one study finding 25% of patients escalated their dosage. Some authors, however, consider benzodiazepines to be effective long-term; however, it is more likely that the drugs are acting to prevent rebound anxiety withdrawal effects. Tolerance to the anticonvulsant and muscle-relaxing effects of benzodiazepines occurs within a few weeks in most patients.[6]

Risk factors

The risk factors for benzodiazepine dependence are long-term use beyond four weeks, use of high doses, use of potent short-acting benzodiazepines, dependent personalities, and proclivity for drug abuse.[14] Use of short-acting benzodiazepines leads to repeated withdrawal effects that are alleviated by the next dose, which reinforce in the individual the dependence.[12] A physical dependence develops more quickly with higher potency benzodiazepines such as alprazolam (Xanax) than with lower potency benzodiazepines such as chlordiazepoxide (Librium).[10]

Symptom severity is worse with the use of high doses, or with benzodiazepines of high potency or short half-life. Other cross-tolerant sedative hypnotics, such as barbiturates or alcohol, increase the risk of benzodiazepine dependence.[15] Similar to opioids' use for pain, therapeutic use of benzodiazepines rarely leads to substance abuse.[16]

2.2.4 Mechanism

Tolerance and physical dependence

See also: Kindling (substance withdrawal)

Tolerance develops rapidly to the sleep-inducing effects of benzodiazepine. The anticonvulsant and muscle-relaxant effects last for a few weeks before tolerance develops in most individuals. Tolerance results in a desensitization of GABA receptors and an increased sensitization of the excitatory neurotransmitter system, glutamate such as NMDA glutamate receptors. These changes occur as a result of the body trying to overcome the drug's effects. Other changes that occur are the reduction of the number of GABA receptors (downregulation) as well as possibly long-term changes in gene transcription coding of brain cells. The differing speed at which tolerance occurs to the therapeutic effects of benzodiazepines can be explained by the speed of changes in the range of neurotransmitter systems and subsystems that are altered by chronic benzodiazepine use. The various neurotransmitter systems and subsystems may reverse tolerance at different speeds, thus explaining the prolonged nature of some withdrawal symptoms. As a result of a physical dependence that develops due to tolerance, a characteristic benzodiazepine withdrawal syndrome often occurs after removal of the drug or a reduction in dosage.[17] Changes in the expression of neuropeptides such as corticotropin-releasing hormone and neuropeptide Y may play a role in benzodiazepine dependence.[18] Individuals taking daily benzodiazepine drugs have a reduced sensitivity to further additional doses of benzodiazepines.[19] Tolerance to benzodiazepines can be demonstrated by injecting diazepam into long-term users. In normal subjects, increases in growth hormone occurs, whereas, in benzodiazepine-tolerant individuals, this effect is blunted.[20]

Animal studies have shown that repeated withdrawal from benzodiazepines leads to increasingly severe withdrawal symptoms, including an increased risk of seizures; this phenomenon is known as kindling. Kindling phenomena are well established for repeated ethanol (alcohol) withdrawal; alcohol has a very similar mechanism of tolerance and withdrawal to benzodiazepines, involving the GABAa, NMDA, and AMPA receptors.[5]

The shift of benzodiazepine receptors to an inverse agonist state after chronic treatment leads the brain to be more sensitive to excitatory drugs or stimuli. Excessive glutamate activity can result in excitotoxicity, which may result in neurodegeneration. The glutamate receptor subtype NMDA is well known for its role in causing excitoneurotoxicity. The glutamate receptor subtype AMPA is believed to play an important role in neuronal kindling as well as excitotoxicity during withdrawal from alcohol as well as benzodiazepines. It is highly possible that NMDA receptors are involved in the tolerance to some effects of benzodiazepines.[5]

Animal studies have found that glutamergic changes as a result of benzodiazepine use are responsible for a delayed withdrawal syndrome, which in mice peaks 3 days after cessation of benzodiazepines. This was demonstrated by the ability to avoid the withdrawal syndrome by the administration of AMPA antagonists. It is believed that different glutamate subreceptors, e.g., NMDA and AMPA, are responsible for different stages/time points of the withdrawal syndrome. NMDA receptors are upregulated in the brain as a result of benzodiazepine tolerance. AMPA receptors are also involved in benzodiazepine tolerance and withdrawal.[5][21][21] A decrease in benzodiazepine binding sites in the brain may also occur as part of benzodiazepine tolerance.[22]

Cross tolerance

Benzodiazepines share a similar mechanism of action with various sedative compounds that act by enhancing the GABAA receptor. *Cross tolerance* means that one drug will alleviate the withdrawal effects of another. It also means that tolerance of one drug will result in tolerance of another similarly-acting drug. Benzodiazepines are often used for this reason to detoxify alcohol-dependent patients and can have life-saving properties in preventing or treating severe life-threatening withdrawal syndromes from alcohol, such as delirium tremens. However, although benzodiazepines can be very useful in the acute detoxification of alcoholics, benzodiazepines in themselves act as positive reinforcers in alcoholics, by increasing the desire for alcohol. Low doses of benzodiazepines were found to significantly increase the level of alcohol consumed in alcoholics.[23] Alcoholics dependent on benzodiazepines should not be abruptly withdrawn but be very slowly withdrawn from benzodiazepines, as over-rapid withdrawal is likely to produce severe anxiety or panic, which is well known for being a relapse risk factor in recovering alcoholics.[24]

There is cross tolerance between alcohol, the benzodiazepines, the barbiturates, the nonbenzodiazepine drugs, and corticosteroids, which all act by enhancing the GABAA receptor's function via modulating the chloride ion channel function of the GABAA receptor.[25][26][27][28][29]

Neuroactive steroids, e.g., progesterone and its active metabolite allopregnanolone, are positive modulators of the GABAA receptor and are cross tolerant with benzodiazepines.[30] The active metabolite of progesterone has been found to enhance the binding of benzodiazepines to the benzodiazepine binding sites on the GABAA receptor.[31] The cross-tolerance between GABAA receptor positive modulators occurs because of the similar mechanism of action and the subunit changes that occur from chronic use from one or more of these compounds in expressed receptor isoforms. Abrupt withdrawal from any of these compounds, e.g., barbiturates, benzodiazepines, alcohol, corticosteroids, neuroactive steroids, and nonbenzodiazepines, precipitate similar withdrawal effects characterized by central nervous system hyper-excitability, resulting in symptoms such as increased seizure susceptibility and anxiety.[32] While many of the neuroactive steroids do not produce full tolerance to their therapeutic effects, cross-tolerance to benzodiazepines still occurs as had been demonstrated between the neuroactive steroid ganaxolone and diazepam. Alterations of levels of neuroactive steroids in the body during the menstrual cycle, menopause, pregnancy, and stressful circumstances can lead to a reduction in the effectiveness of benzodiazepines and a reduced therapeutic effect. During withdrawal of neuroactive steroids, benzodiazepines become less effective.[33]

Physiology of withdrawal

Withdrawal symptoms are a normal response in individuals having chronically used benzodiazepines, and an adverse effect and result of drug tolerance. Symptoms typically emerge when dosage of the drug is reduced. GABA is the second-most-common neurotransmitter in the central nervous system (the most common being glutamate[34][35][36]) and by far the most abundant inhibitory neurotransmitter; roughly one-quarter to one-third of synapses use GABA.[37] The use of benzodiazepines has a profound effect on almost every aspect of brain and body function, either directly or indirectly.[38]

Benzodiazepines cause a decrease in norepinephrine (noradrenaline), serotonin, acetylcholine, and dopamine. These neurotransmitters are needed for normal memory, mood, muscle tone and coordination, emotional responses, endocrine gland secretions, heart rate, and blood pressure control. With chronic benzodiazepine use, tolerance develops rapidly to most of its effects, so that, when benzodiazepines are withdrawn, various neurotransmitter systems go into overdrive due to the lack of inhibitory GABA-ergic activity. Withdrawal symptoms then emerge as a result, and persist until the nervous system physically reverses the adaptions (physical dependence) that have occurred in the CNS.[38]

Withdrawal symptoms typically consist of a mirror image of the drug's effects: Sedative effects and suppression of REM and SWS stages of sleep can be replaced by insomnia, nightmares, and hypnogogic hallucinations; its antianxiety effects are replaced with anxiety and panic; muscle-relaxant effects are replaced with muscular spasms or cramps; and anticonvulsant effects are replaced with seizures, especially in cold turkey or overly-rapid withdrawal.[38]

Benzodiazepine withdrawal represents in part excitotoxicity to brain neurons.[39] Rebound activity of the hypothalamic-pituitary-adrenocortical axis also plays an important role in the severity of benzodiazepine withdrawal.[40] Tolerance and the resultant withdrawal syndrome may be due to alterations in gene expression, which results in long-term changes in the function of the GABAergic neuronal system.[41][42]

During withdrawal from full or partial agonists, changes occur in benzodiazepine receptor with upregulation of some receptor subtypes and downregulation of other receptor subtypes.[43]

Withdrawal

See also: Benzodiazepine withdrawal syndrome

Long-term use of benzodiazepines leads to increasing physical and mental health problems, and as a result, discontinuation is recommended for many long-term users. The withdrawal syndrome from benzodiazepines can range from a mild and short-lasting syndrome to a prolonged and severe syndrome. Withdrawal symptoms can lead to continued use of benzodiazepines for many years, long after the original reason for taking benzodiazepines has passed. Many patients know that the benzodiazepines no longer work for them but are unable to discontinue benzodiazepines because of withdrawal symptoms.[38]

Withdrawal symptoms can emerge despite slow reduction but can be reduced by a slower rate of withdrawal. As a result, withdrawal rates have been recommended to be customized to each individual patient. The time needed to withdrawal can vary from a couple of months to a year or more and often depends on length of use, dosage taken, lifestyle, health, and social and environmental stress factors.[38]

Diazepam is often recommended due to its long elimination half-life and also because of its availability in low potency doses. The non-benzodiazepine Z drugs such as zolpidem, zaleplon, and zopiclone should not be used as a replacement for benzodiazepines, as they have a similar mechanism of action and can induce a similar dependence. The pharmacological mechanism of benzodiazepine tolerance and dependence is the internalization (removal) of receptor site in the brain and changes in gene transcription codes in the brain.[38]

With long-term use and during withdrawal of benzodiazepines, treatment-emergent depression and[6] emotional blunting may emerge and sometimes also suicidal ideation. There is evidence that the higher the dose used the more likely it is benzodiazepine use will induce these feelings. Reducing the dose or discontinuing benzodiazepines may be indicated in such cases. Withdrawal symptoms can persist for quite some time after discontinuing benzodiazepines. Some common protracted withdrawal symptoms include anxiety, depression, insomnia, and physical symptoms such as gastrointestinal, neurologic, and musculoskeletal effects. The protracted withdrawal state may still occur despite slow titration of dosage. It is believed that the protracted withdrawal effects are due to persisting neuroadaptations.[10]

2.2.5 Prevention

Due to the risk of developing tolerance, dependence, and adverse health effects,[44] such as cognitive impairment,[18] benzodiazepines are indicated for short-term use only - a few weeks, followed by a gradual dose reduction.[45]

The Committee on the Review of Medicines (UK)

The Committee on the Review of Medicines carried out a review into benzodiazepines due to significant concerns of tolerance, drug dependence, benzodiazepine withdrawal problems, and other adverse effects and published the results in the British Medical Journal in March 1980. The committee found that benzodiazepines do not have any antidepressant or analgesic properties and are, therefore, unsuitable treatments for conditions such as depression, tension headaches, and dysmenorrhea. Benzodiazepines are also not beneficial in the treatment of psychosis. The committee also recommended against benzodiazepines for use in the treatment of anxiety or insomnia in children.[46]

The committee was in agreement with the Institute of Medicine (USA) and the conclusions of a study carried out by the White House Office of Drug Policy and the National Institute on Drug Abuse (USA) that there is little evidence that long-term use of benzodiazepine hypnotics are beneficial in the treatment of insomnia due to the development of tolerance. Benzodiazepines tend to lose their sleep-promoting properties within 3–14 days of continuous use, and, in the treatment of anxiety, the committee found that there was little convincing evidence that benzodiazepines retains efficacy in the treatment of anxiety after 4 months of continuous use due to the development of tolerance.[46]

The committee found that the regular use of benzodiazepines causes the development of dependence characterized by tolerance to the therapeutic effects of benzodiazepines and the development of the benzodiazepine withdrawal syndrome including symptoms such as anxiety, apprehension, tremors, insomnia, nausea, and vomiting upon cessation of benzodiazepine use. Withdrawal symptoms tend to develop within 24 hours upon cessation of short-acting benzodiazepines, and 3–10 days after cessation of longer-acting benzodiazepines. Withdrawal effects could occur after treatment, lasting only 2 weeks at therapeutic dose levels; however, withdrawal effects tend to occur with habitual use beyond 2 weeks and are more likely the higher the dose. The withdrawal symptoms may appear to be similar to the original condition.[46]

The committee recommended that all benzodiazepine treatment be withdrawn gradually and recommended that benzodiazepine treatment be used only in carefully selected patients and that therapy be limited to short-term use only. It was noted in the review that alcohol can potentiate the central nervous system-depressant effects of benzodiazepines and should be avoided. The central nervous system-depressant effects of benzodiazepines may make driving or operating machinery dangerous, and the elderly are more prone to these adverse effects. High single doses or repeated low doses have been reported to produce hypotonia, poor sucking, and hypothermia in the neonate, and irregularities in the fetal heart. The committee recommended that benzodiazepines be avoided in lactation.[46]

The committee recommended that withdrawal from benzodiazepines be gradual, as abrupt withdrawal from high doses of benzodiazepines may cause confusion, toxic psychosis, convulsions, or a condition resembling delirium tremens. Abrupt withdrawal from lower doses may cause depression, nervousness, rebound insomnia, irritability, sweating, and diarrhea.[46]

The committee also made a mistake concluding:[46]

> on the present available evidence, the true addiction potential of benzodiazepines was low. The number dependant on the benzodiazepines in the UK from 1960 to 1977 has been estimated to be 28 persons. This is equivalent to a dependance rate of 5-10 cases per million patient months.

2.2.6 Diagnosis

For a diagnosis of benzodiazepine dependence to be made, the ICD-10 requires that at least 3 of the below criteria are met and that they have been present for at least a month, or, if less than a month, that they appeared repeatedly during a 12-month period.[47][48]

- Behavioral, cognitive, and physiological phenomena that are associated with the repeated use and that typically include a strong desire to take the drug.

- Difficulty controlling use

- Continued use despite harmful consequences

- Preference given to drug use rather than to other activities and obligations

- Increased tolerance to effects of the drug and sometimes a physical withdrawal state.

These diagnostic criteria are good for research purposes, but, in everyday clinical practice, they should be interpreted according to clinical judgement. In clinical practice, benzodiazepine dependence should be suspected in those having used benzodiazepines for longer than a month, in particular, if they are from a high-risk group. The main factors associated with an increased incidence of benzodiazepine dependence include:[47]

- Dose
- Duration
- Concomitant use of antidepressants

Benzodiazepine dependence should be suspected also in individuals having substance use disorders including alcohol, and should be suspected in individuals obtaining their own supplies of benzodiazepines. Benzodiazepine dependence is almost certain in individuals who are members of a tranquillizer self-help groups.[47]

Research has found that about 40 percent of people with a diagnosis of benzodiazepine dependence are not aware that they are dependent on benzodiazepines, whereas about 11 percent of people judged not to be dependent believe that they are. When assessing a person for benzodiazepine dependence, asking specific questions rather than questions based on concepts is recommended by experts as the best approach of getting a more accurate diagnosis. For example, asking persons if they "think about the medication at times of the day other than when they take the drug" would provide a more meaningful answer than asking "do you think you are psychologically dependent?".[47] The Benzodiazepine Dependence Self Report Questionnaire is one questionnaire used to assess and diagnose benzodiazepine dependence.[47]

2.2.7 In the elderly

See also: Benzodiazepine withdrawal syndrome § Elderly

Long-term use and benzodiazepine dependence is a serious problem in the elderly. Failure to treat benzodiazepine dependence in the elderly can cause serious medical complications.[49] The elderly have less cognitive reserve and are more sensitive to the short (e.g., in between dose withdrawal) and protracted withdrawal effects of benzodiazepines, as well as the side-effects both from short-term and long-term use. This can lead to excessive contact with their doctor. Research has found that withdrawing elderly people from benzodiazepines leads to a significant reduction in doctor visits per year, it is presumed, due to an elimination of drug side-effects and withdrawal effects.[10]

Tobacco and alcohol are the most common substances that elderly people get a dependence on or misuse. The next-most-common substance that elderly people develop a drug dependence to or misuse is benzodiazepines. Drug-induced cognitive problems can have serious consequences for elderly people and can lead to confusional states and "pseudo-dementia". About 10% of elderly patients referred to memory clinics actually have a drug-induced cause that most often is benzodiazepines. Benzodiazepines have also been linked to an increased risk of road traffic accidents and falls in the elderly. The long-term effects of benzodiazepines are still not fully understood in the elderly or any age group. Long-term benzodiazepine use is associated with attentional and visuospatial functional impairments. Withdrawal from benzodiazepines can lead to improved alertness and decreased forgetfulness in the elderly. Withdrawal led to statistical significant improvements in memory function and performance related skills in those having withdrawn successfully from benzodiazepines, whereas those having remained on benzodiazepines experienced worsening symptoms. People having withdrawn from benzodiazepines also felt their sleep was more refreshing, making statements such as "*I feel sharper when I wake up*" or "*I feel better, more awake*", or "*It used to take me an hour to fully wake up.*" This suggests that benzodiazepines may actually make insomnia worse in the elderly.[50]

2.2.8 Treatment and prevention

Benzodiazepines are regarded as a highly addictive drug class.[51] A psychological and physical dependence can develop in as short as a few weeks but may take years to develop in other individuals. Patients wanting to withdraw from benzodiazepines typically receive little advice or support, and such withdrawal should be by small increments over a period of months.[52]

Benzodiazepines are usually prescribed only short-term, as there is little justification for their prescribing long-term.[53] Some doctors however, disagree and believe long-term use beyond 4 weeks is sometimes justified, although there is little data to support this viewpoint.[9] Such viewpoints are a minority in the medical literature.[54]

There is no evidence that "drug holidays" or periods of abstinence reduced the risk of dependence; there is evidence from animal studies that such an approach does not prevent dependence from happening. Use of short-acting benzodiazepines is associated with interdose withdrawal symptoms, which may increase the risk of kindling; kindling has clinical relevance with regard to benzodiazepines; for example, there is an increasing shift to use of benzodiazepines with a shorter half-life and intermittent use, which can result in interdose withdrawal and rebound effects.[5]

Flumazenil as treatment for benzodiazepine dependence

In Italy, the gold standard for treatment of high-dose benzodiazepine dependency is 8–10 days of low dose, slow infusion of flumazenil.[55] One addiction treatment centre in Italy has used flumazenil to treat over 300 patients who are dependent on high doses of benzodiazepines (up to 70 times higher than conventionally prescribed) with doctors being one of their most common patients.[56]

Epileptic patients who have become tolerant to the antiseizure effects of the benzodiazepine clonazepam became seizure-free for several days after treatment with 1.5 mg flumazenil.[57] Similarly, patients who were dependent on high doses of benzodiazepines (median dosage equal to 333 mg diazepam-equivalent) were able to be stabilised on a low dose of clonazepam after 7–8 days of treatment with flumazenil.[58]

Flumazenil has been compared to placebo in dependent subjects, whereby typical benzodiazepine effects were reversed with little to no withdrawal symptoms.[59] Flumazenil was shown to produce significantly less withdrawal symptoms than saline in a randomized, placebo-controlled study with benzodiazepine dependent subjects. Additionally, relapse rates were much less during subsequent follow-up.[60]

Several studies have shown enhancement of the benzodiazepine binding site after chronic treatment with flumazenil where sites have become more numerous and uncoupling/down-regulation of GABAA has been reversed.[61][62][63] After long-term exposure to benzodiazepines, GABAA receptors become down-regulated and uncoupled. Growth of new receptors and recoupling after prolonged flumazenil exposure has also been observed. It is thought this may be due to increased synthesis of receptor proteins.[64]

Flumazenil was found to be more effective than placebo in reducing feelings of hostility and aggression in patients who had been free of benzodiazepines for 4–266 weeks.[65] This may suggest a role for flumazenil in treating protracted benzodiazepine withdrawal symptoms.

Letter to patients

Sending a letter to patients warning of the adverse effects of long-term use of benzodiazepines and recommending dosage reduction has been found to be successful and a cost-effective strategy in reducing benzodiazepine consumption in general practice. Within a year of the letter's going out, there was found to be a 17% fall in the number of benzodiazepines being prescribed, with 5% of patients having totally discontinued benzodiazepines.[66][67] A study in the Netherlands reported a higher success rate by sending a letter to patients who are benzodiazepine-dependent. The results of the Dutch study reported 11.3% of patients discontinuing benzodiazepines completely within a year.[68]

Pharmacist intervention programs

A study found that pharmacists providing educational sessions for medical staff at nursing homes for the elderly combined with medicine audits and feedback cycles combined with an interdisciplinary sedative review resulted in a large reduction in both the number of residents taking benzodiazepines or antipsychotics at all as well as an overall reduction in total dosage.[69]

Cognitive behavioral therapy

Zopiclone is the most frequently prescribed hypnotic in the UK, followed by nitrazepam, and then temazepam, which is the most strictly regulated benzodiazepine in the UK due to its popularity as a drug of abuse and due to its considerably more toxic nature. Hypnotic drugs are of poor value for the management of chronic insomnia. Hypnotic drug consumption has been shown to reduce work performance, increase absenteeism, increase road traffic accidents, increase morbidity, and increase mortality, and is associated with an increased incidence of deliberate self-harm. In the elderly, increases in falls and fractures associated with sedative hypnotic drug use has been found. It is widely accepted that hypnotic drug usage beyond 4 weeks is undesirable for all age groups of patients. Many continuous hypnotic users exhibit disturbed sleep as a consequence of tolerance but experience worsening rebound or withdrawal insomnia when the dose is reduced too quickly, which compounds the problem of chronic hypnotic drug use. Cognitive behavioral therapy has been found to be more effective for the long-term management of insomnia than sedative hypnotic drugs. No formal withdrawal programs for benzodiazepines exists with local providers in the UK. Meta-analysis of published data on psychological treatments for insomnia show a success rate between 70 and 80%. A large-scale trial utilizing cognitive behavioral therapy in chronic users of sedative hypnotics including nitrazepam, temazepam, and zopiclone found CBT to be a significantly more effective long-term treatment for chronic insomnia than sedative hypnotic drugs. Persisting improvements in sleep quality, sleep onset latency, increased total sleep, improvements in sleep efficiency, significant improvements in vitality, physical and mental health at 3-, 6-, and 12-month follow-ups were found in those receiving CBT. A marked reduction in total sedative hypnotic drug use was found in those receiving CBT, with 33% reporting zero hypnotic drug use. Age has been found not to be a barrier to successful outcome of CBT. It was concluded that CBT for the management of chronic insomnia is a flexible, practical, and cost-effective treatment, and it was also concluded that CBT leads to a reduction of benzodiazepine drug intake in a significant number of patients.[70] Chronic use of hypnotic medications is not recommended due to their adverse effects on health and the risk of dependence. A gradual taper is usual clinical course in getting people off of benzodiazepines, but, even with gradual reduction, a large proportion of people fail to stop taking benzodiazepines. The elderly are particularly sensitive to the adverse effects of hypnotic medications. A clinical trial in elderly people dependent on benzodiazepine hypnotics showed that the addition of CBT to a gradual benzodiazepine reduction program increased the success rate of discontinuing benzodiazepine hypnotic drugs from 38% to 77% and at the 12-month follow-up from 24% to 70%. The paper concluded that CBT is an effective tool for reducing hypnotic use in the elderly and reducing the adverse health effects that are associated with hypnotics such as drug dependence, cognitive impairments, and increased road traffic accidents.[71]

A study of patients undergoing benzodiazepine withdrawal who had a diagnosis of generalized anxiety disorder showed that those having received CBT had a very high success rate of discontinuing benzodiazepines compared to those not having receive CBT. This success rate was maintained at the 12-month follow-up. Furthermore, it was found that, in patients having discontinued benzodiazepines, they no longer met the diagnosis of general anxiety disorder, and that the number of patients no longer meeting the diagnosis of general anxiety disorder was higher in the group having received CBT. Thus, CBT can be an effective tool to add to a gradual benzodiazepine dosage reduction program leading to improved and sustained mental health benefits.[72]

Legal implications

Negligent management of the benzodiazepine withdrawal syndrome has led to some doctors' being brought before the General Medical Council in the UK, for example, for stopping sleeping tablets abruptly or reducing anxiolytics too quickly, failure to initiate replacement therapy (e.g., equivalent dose of diazepam), failure to increase dosage to alleviate severe withdrawal effects, and failure to warn the patient of the possibility of withdrawal symptoms, having led to a finding by the GMC of negligence against one doctor.[73]

2.2.9 Epidemiology

Research studies have come to different conclusions on the number of therapeutic dose users who develop a physical dependence and withdrawal syndrome. Estimates by researchers of the number of people affected range 20–100% of patients prescribed benzodiazepines at therapeutic dosages long term are physically dependent and will experience withdrawal symptoms.[74]

Benzodiazepines can be addictive and induce dependence even at low doses, with 23% becoming addicted within 3 months of use. Benzodiazepine addiction is considered a public health problem. Approximately 68.5% of prescriptions of benzodiazepines originate from local health centers, with psychiatry and general hospitals accounting for 10% each. A survey of general practitioners reported that the reason for initiating benzodiazepines was due to an empathy for the patients suffering and a lack of other therapeutic options rather than patients demanding them. However, long-term use was more commonly at the insistence of the patient, it is presumed, because physical dependence or addiction had developed.[75][76][77]

Approximately twice as many women as men are prescribed benzodiazepines. It is believed that this is largely because men typically turned to alcohol to cope with stress and women to prescription drugs. Biased perception of women by male doctors may also play a role in increased prescribing rates to women; however, increased anxiety features in women does not account for the wide gap alone between men and women.[20]

2.2.10 History

Previously, physical dependence on benzodiazepines was largely thought to occur only in people on high-therapeutic-dose ranges and low- or normal-dose dependence was not suspected until the 1970s; and it was not until the early 1980s that it was confirmed.[78][79] Low-dose dependence has now been clearly demonstrated in both animal studies and human studies,[80][81] and is a recognized clinical disadvantage of benzodiazepines. Severe withdrawal syndromes can occur from these low doses of benzodiazepines even after gradual dose reduction.[82][83] An estimated 30–45% of chronic low-dose benzodiazepine users are dependent and it has been recommended that benzodiazepines even at low dosage be prescribed for a maximum of 7–14 days to avoid dependence.[84] As a result, strict regulations for the prescription of benzodiazepines due to this risk of low-dose dependence.[85]

Some controversy remains, however, in the medical literature as to the exact nature of low-dose dependence and the difficulty in getting patients to discontinue their benzodiazepines, with some papers attributing the problem to predominantly drug-seeking behavior and drug craving, whereas other papers having found the opposite, attributing the problem to a problem of physical dependence with drug-seeking and craving not being typical of low-dose benzodiazepine users.[86][87]

2.2.11 Misuse and addiction

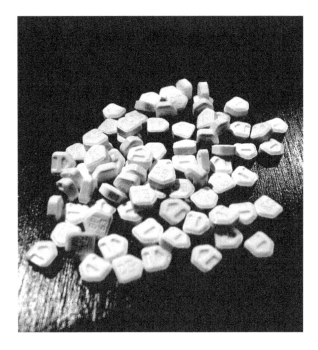

Lorazepam (Ativan) tablets.

See also: Benzodiazepine misuse

Benzodiazepines are one of the largest classes of abused drugs; they are classed as schedule IV controlled drugs because of their recognized medical uses.[88] Across the world the most frequently diverted and abused benzodiazepines include temazepam, diazepam, nimetazepam, nitrazepam, triazolam, flunitrazepam, midazolam, and in the United States alprazolam, clonazepam, and lorazepam.

Benzodiazepines can cause serious addiction problems. A survey in Senegal of doctors found that many doctors feel that their training and knowledge of benzodiazepines is, in general, poor; a study in Dakar found that almost one-fifth of doctors ignored prescribing guidelines regarding short-term use of benzodiazepines, and almost three-quarters of doctors regarded their training and knowledge of benzodiazepines to be inadequate. More training regarding benzodiazepines has been recommended for doctors.[89] Due to the serious concerns of addiction, national governments were recommended to urgently seek to raise knowledge via training about the addictive nature of benzodiazepines and appropriate prescribing of benzodiazepines.[90]

A six-year study on 51 Vietnam veterans who were drug abusers of either mainly stimulants (11 people), mainly opiates (26 people), or mainly benzodiazepines (14 people) was carried out to assess psychiatric symptoms related to the specific drugs of abuse. After six years, opiate abusers had little change in psychiatric symptomatology; five of the stimulant users had developed psychosis, and eight of the benzodiazepine users had developed depression. Therefore, long-term benzodiazepine abuse and dependence seems to carry a negative effect on mental health, with a significant risk of causing depression.[91] Benzodiazepines are also sometimes abused intra-nasally.[92]

In the elderly, alcohol and benzodiazepines are the most commonly abused substances, and the elderly population is more susceptible to benzodiazepine withdrawal syndrome and delirium than are younger patients.[93]

2.2.12 See also

- Long-term effects of benzodiazepines
- Alcohol withdrawal syndrome
- Long-term effects of alcohol
- SSRI discontinuation syndrome
- Drug related crime

2.2.13 References

[1] de Wit H; Griffiths RR (June 1991). "Testing the abuse liability of anxiolytic and hypnotic drugs in humans". *Drug and Alcohol Dependence* **28** (1): 83–111. doi:10.1016/0376-8716(91)90054-3. PMID 1679388. Retrieved 21 December 2012.

[2] Nutt DJ (1 January 1986). "Benzodiazepine dependence in the clinic: reason for anxiety". *Trends neurosci* **7**: 457–460. doi:10.1016/0165-6147(86)90420-7. Retrieved 21 December 2012.

[3] Uzun S; Kozumplik O; Jakovljević M; Sedić B (Mar 2010). "Side effects of treatment with benzodiazepines". *Psychiatr Danub* **22** (1): 90–3. PMID 20305598.

[4] O'brien CP (2005). "Benzodiazepine use, abuse, and dependence". *J Clin Psychiatry* **66** (Suppl 2): 28–33. PMID 15762817.

[5] Allison C; Pratt JA (May 2003). "Neuroadaptive processes in GABAergic and glutamatergic systems in benzodiazepine dependence". *Pharmacol. Ther.* **98** (2): 171–95. doi:10.1016/S0163-7258(03)00029-9. PMID 12725868.

[6] Haddad P; Deakin B; Dursun S (27 May 2004). "Benzodiazepine dependence". *Adverse Syndromes and Psychiatric Drugs: A clinical guide*. Oxford University Press. pp. 240–252. ISBN 978-0-19-852748-0.

[7] Cloos JM; Ferreira V (January 2009). "Current use of benzodiazepines in anxiety disorders". *Current Opinion in Psychiatry* **22** (1): 90–95. doi:10.1097/YCO.0b013e32831a473d. PMID 19122540.

[8] Licata SC; Rowlett JK (2008). "Abuse and dependence liability of benzodiazepine-type drugs: GABA(A) receptor modulation and beyond.". *Pharmacology Biochemistry and Behavior* **90** (1): 74–89. doi:10.1016/j.pbb.2008.01.001. PMC 2453238. PMID 18295321.

[9] Puri BK; Tyrer P (28 August 1998). "Clinical psychopharmacology". *Sciences Basic to Psychiatry* (2nd ed.). Churchill Livingstone. pp. 155–157. ISBN 978-0-443-05514-0. Retrieved 2009-07-11.

[10] Longo LP; Johnson B (April 2000). "Addiction: Part I. Benzodiazepines--side effects, abuse risk and alternatives". *Am Fam Physician* **61** (7): 2121–8. PMID 10779253.

[11] Authier=N; Balayssac D; Sautereau M; Zangarelli A; Courty P; Somogyi AA; Vennat B; Llorca PM; Eschalier A (Nov 2009). "Benzodiazepine dependence: focus on withdrawal syndrome". *Ann Pharm Fr* **67** (6): 408–13. doi:10.1016/j.pharma.2009.07.001. PMID 19900604.

[12] Khong E; Sim MG; Hulse G (Nov 2004). "Benzodiazepine dependence" (PDF). *Aust Fam Physician* **33** (11): 923–6. PMID 15584332.

[13] National Treatment Agency for Substance Misuse (2007). "Drug misuse and dependence - UK guidelines on clinical management" (PDF). United Kingdom: Department of Health.

[14] Marriott S; Tyrer P (August 1993). "Benzodiazepine dependence. Avoidance and withdrawal". *Drug safety: an international journal of medical toxicology and drug experience.* **9** (2): 93–103. doi:10.2165/00002018-199309020-00003. PMID 8104417.

[15] Pétursson H (1994). "The benzodiazepine withdrawal syndrome". *Addiction* **89** (11): 1455–9. doi:10.1111/j.1360-0443.1994.tb03743.x. PMID 7841856.

[16] Galanter M; Kleber HD (1 July 2008). *The American Psychiatric Publishing Textbook of Substance Abuse Treatment* (4th ed.). United States of America: American Psychiatric Publishing Inc. p. 114. ISBN 978-1-58562-276-4.

[17] Ashton H (2005). "The diagnosis and management of benzodiazepine dependence" (PDF). *Current Opinion in Psychiatry* **18** (3): 249–55. doi:10.1097/01.yco.0000165594.60434.84. PMID 16639148.

[18] Heberlein A; Bleich S; Kornhuber J; Hillemacher T (Jan 2009). "[Benzodiazepine dependence: causalities and treatment options]". *Fortschr Neurol Psychiatr* **77** (1): 7–15. doi:10.1055/s-0028-1100831. PMID 19101875.

[19] Potokar J; Coupland N; Wilson S; Rich A; Nutt D (September 1999). "Assessment of GABA(A)benzodiazepine receptor (GBzR) sensitivity in patients on benzodiazepines". *Psychopharmacology (Berl.)* **146** (2): 180–4. doi:10.1007/s002130051104. PMID 10525753.

[20] Lader Prof; Morgan Prof; Shepherd Prof; Williams Dr P; Skegg Dr; Parish Prof; Tyrer Dr P; Inman Dr; Marks Dr J (Ex-Roche); Harris P (Roche); Hurry T (Wyeth) (30 October 1980 – 3 April 1981). "Benzodiazepine Dependence Medical Research Council headquarters, Closed until 2014 - Opened 2005" (PDF). England: The National Archives.

[21] Koff JM; Pritchard GA; Greenblatt DJ; Miller LG (November 1997). "The NMDA receptor competitive antagonist CPP modulates benzodiazepine tolerance and discontinuation". *Pharmacology* **55** (5): 217–27. doi:10.1159/000139531. PMID 9399331.

[22] Fujita M; Woods SW; Verhoeff NP; et al. (March 1999). "Changes of benzodiazepine receptors during chronic benzodiazepine administration in humans". *Eur. J. Pharmacol.* **368** (2–3): 161–72. doi:10.1016/S0014-2999(99)00013-8. PMID 10193652.

[23] Poulos CX; Zack M (2004). "Low-dose diazepam primes motivation for alcohol and alcohol-related semantic networks in problem drinkers". *Behavioural Pharmacology* **15** (7): 503–12. doi:10.1097/00008877-200411000-00006. PMID 15472572.

[24] Kushner MG; Abrams K; Borchardt C (March 2000). "The relationship between anxiety disorders and alcohol use disorders: a review of major perspectives and findings". *Clin Psychol Rev* **20** (2): 149–71. doi:10.1016/S0272-7358(99)00027-6. PMID 10721495.

[25] Khanna JM; Kalant H; Weiner J; Shah G (1992). "Rapid tolerance and cross-tolerance as predictors of chronic tolerance and cross-tolerance". *Pharmacol. Biochem. Behav.* **41** (2): 355–60. doi:10.1016/0091-3057(92)90110-2. PMID 1574525.

[26] World Health Organisation - Assessment of Zopiclone

[27] Allan AM; Baier LD; Zhang X (1992). "Effects of lorazepam tolerance and withdrawal on GABAA receptor-operated chloride channels". *J. Pharmacol. Exp. Ther.* **261** (2): 395–402. PMID 1374467.

[28] Rooke KC (1976). "The use of flurazepam (dalmane) as a substitute for barbiturates and methaqualone/diphenhydramine (mandrax) in general practice". *J Int Med Res* **4** (5): 355–9. doi:10.1177/030006057600400510. PMID 18375.

[29] Reddy DS; Rogawski MA (1 December 2000). "Chronic treatment with the neuroactive steroid ganaxolone in the rat induces anticonvulsant tolerance to diazepam but not to itself". *J Pharmacol Exp Ther* **295** (3): 1241–8. PMID 11082461.

[30] Martin D; Olsen RW (2000). *GABA in the nervous system: the view at fifty*. Philadelphia: Lippincott Williams Wilkins. p. 211. ISBN 0-7817-2267-5.

[31] Kroboth PD; McAuley JW (1997). "Progesterone: does it affect response to drug?". *Psychopharmacol Bull* **33** (2): 297–301. PMID 9230647.

[32] Smith SS (2004). *Neurosteroid effects in the central nervous system: the role of the GABA-A receptor*. Boca Raton, Fla.: CRC Press. pp. 144–145. ISBN 978-0-8493-2392-8.

[33] Rho JM; Sankar R; Cavazos JE (2004). *Epilepsy: scientific foundations of clinical practice*. New York: M. Dekker. p. 336. ISBN 978-0-8247-5043-5.

[34] Kaltschmidt C; Kaltschmidt B; Baeuerle PA (1995). "Stimulation of ionotropic glutamate receptors activates transcription factor NF-kappa B in primary neurons". *Proc. Natl. Acad. Sci. U.S.A.* **92** (21): 9618–22. doi:10.1073/pnas.92.21.9618. PMC 40853. PMID 7568184.

[35] Humphries P; Pretorius E; Naudé H (2007). "Direct and indirect cellular effects of aspartame on the brain". *European Journal of Clinical Nutrition* **62** (4): 451–62. doi:10.1038/sj.ejcn.1602866. ISSN 0954-3007. PMID 17684524.

[36] Herlenius E, Langercrantz H (2004). "Development of neurotransmitter systems during critical periods". *Exp Neurol* **190**: 8–21. doi:10.1016/j.expneurol.2004.03.027.

[37] "Synapses". *The Brain from Top to Bottom*. McGill University.

[38] Professor Heather Ashton (2002). "Benzodiazepines: How They Work and How to Withdraw".

[39] Brown TM; Stoudemire (1998). "Chapter 7 Sedative-Hypnotics and Related Agents". *Psychiatric side effects of prescription and over-the-counter medications: recognition and management*. USA: American Psychiatric Press Inc. pp. 132–133. ISBN 0-88048-868-9.

[40] Wichniak A; Brunner H; Ising M; Pedrosa Gil F; Holsboer F; Friess E (October 2004). "Impaired hypothalamic-pituitary-adrenocortical (HPA) system is related to severity of benzodiazepine withdrawal in patients with depression". *Psychoneuroendocrinology* **29** (9): 1101–8. doi:10.1016/j.psyneuen.2003.11.004. PMID 15219633.

[41] Biggio G; Dazzi L; Biggio F; et al. (December 2003). "Molecular mechanisms of tolerance to and withdrawal of GABA(A) receptor modulators". *Eur Neuropsychopharmacol* **13** (6): 411–23. doi:10.1016/j.euroneuro.2003.08.002. PMID 14636957.

[42] Bateson AN (2002). "Basic pharmacologic mechanisms involved in benzodiazepine tolerance and withdrawal". *Curr. Pharm. Des.* **8** (1): 5–21. doi:10.2174/1381612023396681. PMID 11812247.

[43] Follesa P; Cagetti E; Mancuso L; et al. (August 2001). "Increase in expression of the GABA(A) receptor alpha(4) subunit gene induced by withdrawal of, but not by long-term treatment with, benzodiazepine full or partial agonists". *Brain Res. Mol. Brain Res.* **92** (1–2): 138–48. doi:10.1016/S0169-328X(01)00164-4. PMID 11483250.

[44] Tyrer P; Silk KR, eds. (24 January 2008). "Treatment of sedative-hypnotic dependence". *Cambridge Textbook of Effective Treatments in Psychiatry* (1st ed.). Cambridge University Press. p. 402. ISBN 978-0-521-84228-0.

[45] Karch SB (20 December 2006). *Drug Abuse Handbook* (2nd ed.). United States of America: CRC Press. p. 617. ISBN 978-0-8493-1690-6.

[46] Committee on the Review of Medicines (March 29, 1980). "Systematic review of the benzodiazepines. Guidelines for data sheets on diazepam, chlordiazepoxide, medazepam, clorazepate, lorazepam, oxazepam, temazepam, triazolam, nitrazepam, and flurazepam. Committee on the Review of Medicines". *Br Med J* **280** (6218): 910–2. doi:10.1136/bmj.280.6218.910. PMC 1601049. PMID 7388368.

[47] Polmear A (31 March 2008). *Evidence-Based Diagnosis in Primary Care: Practical Solutions to Common Problems*. United Kingdom: Butterworth-Heinemann. pp. 346–347. ISBN 978-0-7506-4910-0.

[48] ICD-10 (2007). "Chapter V - Mental and behavioural disorders (F00-F99) - Mental and behavioural disorders due to psychoactive substance use, 10-F19)". World Health Organisation. Archived from the original on 2009-07-27.

[49] Madhusoodanan S; Bogunovic OJ (September 2004). "Safety of benzodiazepines in the geriatric population". *Expert Opin Drug Saf* **3** (5): 485–93. doi:10.1517/14740338.3.5.485. PMID 15335303.

[50] Baillargeon L; Landreville P; Verreault R; Beauchemin JP; Grégoire JP; Morin CM (November 2003). "Discontinuation of benzodiazepines among older insomniac adults treated with cognitive-behavioural therapy combined with gradual tapering: a randomized trial" (PDF). *CMAJ* **169** (10): 1015–20. PMC 236226. PMID 14609970.

[51] Casati A; Sedefov R; Pfeiffer-Gerschel T (2012). "Misuse of medicines in the European Union: a systematic review of the literature" (PDF). *Eur Addict Res* **18** (5): 228–45. doi:10.1159/000337028. PMID 22572594.

[52] Authier N; Balayssac D; Sautereau M; Zangarelli A; Courty P; Somogyi AA; Vennat B; Llorca PM; EschalierA (Nov 2009). "Benzodiazepine dependence: focus on withdrawal syndrome". *Ann Pharm Fr* **67** (6): 408–13. doi:10.1016/j.pharma.2009.07.001. PMID 19900604.

[53] Panus P; Katzung BG; Jobst EE; Tinsley S; Masters SB; Trevor AJ (November 2008). "Sedative-hypnotic drugs". *Pharmacology for the Physical Therapist* (1 ed.). McGraw-Hill Medical. p. 192. ISBN 978-0-07-146043-9.

[54] Tyrer P; Silk KR, eds. (24 January 2008). *Cambridge Textbook of Effective Treatments in Psychiatry* (1st ed.). Cambridge University Press. p. 532. ISBN 978-0-521-84228-0.

[55] Lugoboni F; Faccini M; Quaglio G; Casari R; Albiero A; Pajusco B (2011). "Agonist substitution for high-dose benzodiazepine-dependent patients: let us not forget the importance of flumazenil". *Addiction* **106** (4): 853–853. doi:10.1111/j.1360-0443.2010.03327.x. ISSN 0965-2140.

[56] Lugoboni F; Leone R (2012). "What is stopping us from using Flumazenil?". *Addiction* **107** (7): 1359–1359. doi:10.1111/j.1360-0443.2012.03851.x. ISSN 0965-2140.

[57] Savic I (1991). "Feasibility of reversing benzodiazepine tolerance with flumazenil". *The Lancet* **337** (8734): 133–137. doi:10.1016/0140-6736(91)90799-U. ISSN 0140-6736.

[58] Quaglio G; Pattaro C; Gerra G; Mathew S; Verbanck P; Des Jarlais DC; Lugoboni F (2012). "High dose benzodiazepine dependence: Description of 29 patients treated with flumazenil infusion and stabilised with clonazepam". *Psychiatry Research* **198** (3): 457–462. doi:10.1016/j.psychres.2012.02.008. ISSN 0165-1781. PMID 22424905.

[59] Gerra G; Giucasto G; Zaimovic A; Fertonani G; Chittolini B; Avanzini P; Caccavari R (June 1996). "Intravenous flumazenil following prolonged exposure to lormetazepam in humans: lack of precipitated withdrawal". *International clinical psychopharmacology* **11** (2): 81–88. doi:10.1097/00004850-199611020-00002. PMID 8803645.

[60] Gerra G; Zaimovic A; Giusti F; Moi G; Brewer C (2002). "Intravenous flumazenil versus oxazepam tapering in the treatment of benzodiazepine withdrawal: a randomized, placebo-controlled study". *Addiction Biology* **7** (4): 385–395. doi:10.1080/1355621021000005973. ISSN 1355-6215. PMID 14578014.

[61] Pericic D; Lazic J (August 2005). "Chronic treatment with flumazenil enhances binding sites for convulsants at recombinant alpha(1)beta(2)gamma(2S) GABA(A) receptors". *Biomedicine & pharmacotherapy=Biomedecine & pharmacotherapie* **59** (7): 408–414. doi:10.1016/j.biopha.2005.02.003. PMID 16084060.

[62] Pericic D; Jembrek MJ; Strac DS; Lazic J (January 2005). "Enhancement of benzodiazepine binding sites following chronic treatment with flumazenil". *European journal of pharmacology* **507** (1–3): 7–13. doi:10.1016/j.ejphar.2004.10.057. PMID 15659288.

[63] Pericic D; Lazic J; Jembrek MJ; Strac DS (December 2004). "Chronic exposure of cells expressing recombinant GABAA receptors to benzodiazepine antagonist flumazenil enhances the maximum number of benzodiazepine binding sites". *Life sciences* **76** (3): 303–317. doi:10.1016/j.lfs.2004.07.013. PMID 15531382.

[64] Jembrek MJ; Strac DS; Vlainic J (July 2008). "The role of transcriptional and translational mechanisms in flumazenil-induced up-regulation of recombinant GABA(A) receptors". *Neuroscience research* **61** (3): 234–241. doi:10.1016/j.neures.2008.03.005. PMID 18453026.

[65] Saxon L; Borg S (August 2010). "Reduction of aggression during benzodiazepine withdrawal: effects of flumazenil". *Pharmacology, biochemistry, and behavior* **96** (2): 148–151. doi:10.1016/j.pbb.2010.04.023. PMID 20451546.

[66] Morgan JD; Wright DJ; Chrystyn H (December 2002). "Pharmacoeconomic evaluation of a patient education letter aimed at reducing long-term prescribing of benzodiazepines" (PDF). *Pharm World Sci* **24** (6): 231–5. doi:10.1023/A:1021587209529. PMID 12512155.

[67] Stewart R; Niessen WJ; Broer J; Snijders TA; Haaijer-Ruskamp FM; Meyboom-De Jong B (October 2007). "General Practitioners reduced benzodiazepine prescriptions in an intervention study: a multilevel application". *J Clin Epidemiol* **60** (10): 1076–84. doi:10.1016/j.jclinepi.2006.11.024. PMID 17884604.

[68] Niessen WJ; Stewart RE; Broer J; Haaijer-Ruskamp FM (February 2005). "Vermindering van gebruik van benzodiazepinen door een brief van de eigen huisarts aan chronische gebruikers" [Reduction in the consumption of benzodiazepines due to a letter to chronic users from their own general practitioner]. *Ned Tijdschr Geneeskd* (in Dutch and Flemish) **149** (7): 356–61. PMID 15751808.

[69] Westbury J; Jackson S; Gee P; Peterson G (Oct 2009). "An effective approach to decrease antipsychotic and benzodiazepine use in nursing homes: the RedUSe project". *Int Psychogeriatr* **22** (1): 1–11. doi:10.1017/S1041610209991128. PMID 19814843.

[70] Morgan K; Dixon S; Mathers N; Thompson J; Tomeny M (February 2004). "Psychological treatment for insomnia in the regulation of long-term hypnotic drug use" (PDF). *Health Technol Assess* (National Institute for Health Research) **8** (8): 1–68. doi:10.3310/hta8080. PMID 14960254.

[71] Baillargeon L; Landreville P; Verreault R; Beauchemin JP; Grégoire JP; Morin CM (November 2003). "Discontinuation of benzodiazepines among older insomniac adults treated with cognitive-behavioural therapy combined with gradual tapering: a randomized trial". *CMAJ* **169** (10): 1015–20. PMC 236226. PMID 14609970.

[72] Gosselin P; Ladouceur R; Morin CM; Dugas MJ; Baillargeon L (October 2006). "Benzodiazepine discontinuation among adults with GAD: A randomized trial of cognitive-behavioral therapy". *J Consult Clin Psychol* **74** (5): 908–19. doi:10.1037/0022-006X.74.5.908. PMID 17032095.

[73] Gandy A; Widdup J; Gupta R; Shend'ge E; Popat A (11–15 May 2009). "Fitness to Practice Panel 11–15 May 2009" (PDF). United Kingdom: gmc-uk. Archived from the original (PDF) on 2009.

[74] Ashton CH (1997). "Benzodiazepine Dependency". In Baum A; Newman S; Weinman J; West R; McManus C. *Cambridge Handbook of Psychology & Medicine*. England: Cambridge University Press. pp. 376–80.

[75] Anthierens S; Habraken H; Petrovic M; Christiaens T (December 2007). "The lesser evil? Initiating a benzodiazepine prescription in general practice: a qualitative study on GPs' perspectives" (PDF). *Scand J Prim Health Care* **25** (4): 214–9. doi:10.1080/02813430701726335. PMC 3379762. PMID 18041658.

[76] Granados Menéndez MI; Salinero Fort MA; Palomo Ancillo M; Aliaga Gutiérrez L; García Escalonilla C; Ortega Orcos R (2006). "Adecuacion del uso de las benzodiacepinas zolpidem y zopiclona en problemas atendidos en atencion primaria" [Appropriate use of benzodiazepines zolpidem and zopiclone in diseases attended in primary care]. *Aten Primaria* (in Spanish) **38** (3): 159–64. doi:10.1157/13090980. PMID 16945275.

[77] Barthelmé B; Poirot Y (November 2008). "Niveau d'anxiete et de dependance des primoconsommants d'anxiolytiques: une etude de psychometrie" [Anxiety level and addiction to first-time prescriptions of anxiolytics: a psychometric study]. *Presse Med [Medical Press]* (in French) **37** (11): 1555–60. doi:10.1016/j.lpm.2007.10.019. PMID 18502091.

[78] Fruensgaard K (February 1976). "Withdrawal psychosis: a study of 30 consecutive cases". *Acta Psychiatr Scand* **53** (2): 105–18. doi:10.1111/j.1600-0447.1976.tb00065.x. PMID 3091.

[79] Lader M (1991). "History of benzodiazepine dependence". *Journal of substance abuse treatment* **8** (1–2): 53–9. doi:10.1016/0740-5472(91)90027-8. PMID 1675692.

[80] Lucki I; Kucharik RF (1990). "Increased sensitivity to benzodiazepine antagonists in rats following chronic treatment with a low dose of diazepam". *Psychopharmacology* **102** (3): 350–6. doi:10.1007/BF02244103. PMID 1979180.

[81] Rickels K; Case WG; Schweizer EE; Swenson C; Fridman RB (1986). "Low-dose dependence in chronic benzodiazepine users: a preliminary report on 119 patients". *Psychopharmacology bulletin* **22** (2): 407–15. PMID 2877472.

[82] Lader M (December 1987). "Long-term anxiolytic therapy: the issue of drug withdrawal". *The Journal of clinical psychiatry* **48**: 12–6. PMID 2891684.

[83] Miura S; Murasaki M (March 1992). "The future of 5-HT1A receptor agonists. (Aryl-piperazine derivatives)". *Progress in neuro-psychopharmacology & biological psychiatry* **16** (6): 833–45. doi:10.1016/0278-5846(92)90103-L. PMID 1355301.

[84] Meier PJ; Ziegler WH; Neftel K (March 19, 1988). "Benzodiazepine--Praxis und Probleme ihrer Anwendung" [Benzodiazepine--practice and problems of its use]. *Schweizerische medizinische Wochenschrift [Swiss medical weekly]* **118** (11): 381–92. PMID 3287602.

[85] Tsuji K; Tajima O (January 2012). "[Anxiolytic]". *Nippon Rinsho* (in Japanese) **70** (1): 42–6. PMID 22413490.

[86] Linden M; Bär T; Geiselmann B (May 1998). "Patient treatment insistence and medication craving in long-term low-dosage benzodiazepine prescriptions". *Psychological Medicine* **28** (3): 721–9. doi:10.1017/S0033291798006734. PMID 9626728.

[87] Tyrer P (1993). "Benzodiazepine dependence: a shadowy diagnosis". *Biochemical Society Symposia* **59**: 107–19. PMID 7910738.

[88] Karch SB (20 December 2006). *Drug Abuse Handbook* (2nd ed.). USA: CRC Press. p. 35. ISBN 978-0-8493-1690-6.

[89] Dièye AM; Sy AN; Sy GY; et al. (2007). "Prescription des benzodiazepines par les medecins generalistes du prive a Dakar: Enquete sur les connaissances et les attitudes" [Prescription of benzodiazepines by general practitioners in the private sector of Dakar: survey on knowledge and attitudes]. *Therapie [Therapy]* (in French) **62** (2): 163–8. doi:10.2515/therapie:2007018. PMID 17582318.

[90] Dièye AM; Sylla M; Ndiaye A; Ndiaye M; Sy GY; Faye B (June 2006). "Benzodiazepines prescription in Dakar: a study about prescribing habits and knowledge in general practitioners, neurologists and psychiatrists". *Fundam Clin Pharmacol* **20** (3): 235–8. doi:10.1111/j.1472-8206.2006.00400.x. PMID 16671957.

[91] Woody GE; Mc Lellan AT; O'Brien CP (1979). "Development of psychiatric illness in drug abusers. Possible role of drug preference". *The New England Journal of Medicine* **301** (24): 1310–4. doi:10.1056/NEJM197912133012403. PMID 41182.

[92] Sheehan MF; Sheehan DV; Torres A; Coppola A; Francis E (1991). "Snorting benzodiazepines". *Am J Drug Alcohol Abuse* **17** (4): 457–68. doi:10.3109/00952999109001605. PMID 1684083.

[93] Wetterling T; Backhaus J; Junghanns K (September 2002). "Sucht im Alter Ein unterschätztes Problem in der klinischen Versorgung älterer Menschen?" [Addiction in the elderly - an underestimated diagnosis in clinical practice?]. *Nervenarzt* (in German) **73** (9): 861–6. doi:10.1007/s00115-002-1359-3. PMID 12215877.

2.2.14 External links

- Benzodiazepines: How they work and how to withdraw by Professor Heather Ashton

- Benzodiazepine dependence at DMOZ

2.3 Benzodiazepine withdrawal syndrome

Benzodiazepine withdrawal syndrome—often abbreviated to **benzo withdrawal**—is the cluster of symptoms that emerge when a person who has taken benzodiazepines, either medically or recreationally, and has developed a physical dependence undergoes dosage reduction or discontinuation. Development of physical dependence and or addiction and the resulting withdrawal symptoms, some of which may last for years, may result from either drug seeking behaviors or from taking the medication as prescribed. Benzodiazepine withdrawal is characterized by sleep disturbance, irritability, increased tension and anxiety, panic attacks, hand tremor, sweating, difficulty with concentration, confusion and cognitive difficulty, memory problems, dry retching and nausea, weight loss, palpitations, headache, muscular pain and stiffness, a host of perceptual changes, hallucinations, seizures, psychosis,[1] and suicide[2] (see "Signs and Symptoms" section below for full list). Further, these symptoms are notable for the manner in which they wax and wane and vary in severity from day to day or week by week instead of steadily decreasing in a straightforward monotonic manner.[3]

It is a potentially serious condition, and is complex and often protracted in time course.[4][5] Long-term use, defined as daily use for at least three months,[6] is not desirable because of the associated increased risk of dependence,[7] dose escalation, loss of efficacy, increased risk of accidents and falls, particularly for the elderly,[8] as well as cognitive,[9] neurological, and intellectual impairments.[10] Use of short-acting hypnotics, while being effective at initiating sleep, worsen the second half of sleep due to withdrawal effects.[11] Nevertheless, long-term users of benzodiazepines should not be forced to withdraw against their will.[4]

Benzodiazepine withdrawal can be severe and can provoke life-threatening withdrawal symptoms, such as seizures,[12] particularly with abrupt or overly-rapid dosage reduction from high doses or long time users.[4] A severe withdrawal response can nevertheless occur despite gradual dose reduction, or from relatively low doses in short time users,[13] even after a single large dose in animal models.[14][15] A minority of individuals will experience a protracted withdrawal syndrome whose symptoms may persist at a subacute level for months, or years after cessation of benzodiazepines. The likelihood of developing a protracted withdrawal syndrome can be minimized by a slow, gradual reduction in dosage.[16]

Chronic exposure to benzodiazepines causes neural adaptations that counteract the drug's effects, leading to tolerance and dependence.[17] Despite taking a constant therapeutic dose, long-term use of benzodiazepines may lead to the emergence of withdrawal-like symptoms, particularly between doses.[18] When the drug is discontinued or the dosage reduced, withdrawal symptoms may appear and remain until the body reverses the physiological adaptations.[19] These rebound symptoms may be identical to the symptoms for which the drug was initially taken, or may be part of discontinuation symptoms.[20] In severe cases, the withdrawal reaction may exacerbate or resemble serious psychiatric and medical conditions, such as mania, schizophrenia, and, especially at high doses, seizure disorders.[21] Failure to recognize discontinuation symptoms can lead to false evidence for the need to take benzodiazepines, which in turn leads to withdrawal failure and reinstatement of benzodiazepines, often to higher doses.[21]

Awareness of the withdrawal reactions, individualized taper strategies according to withdrawal severity, the addition of alternative strategies such as reassurance and referral to benzodiazepine withdrawal support groups, all increase the success rate of withdrawal.[22][23]

2.3.1 Signs and symptoms

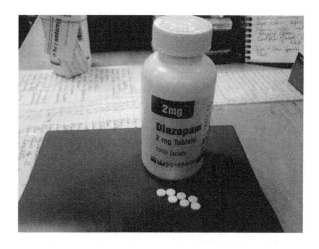

Diazepam, 2 mg and 5 mg diazepam tablets, are commonly used in the treatment of benzodiazepine withdrawal.

Withdrawal effects caused by sedative-hypnotics discontinuation, such as benzodiazepines, barbiturates, or alcohol, can cause serious medical complications. They are cited to be more hazardous to withdraw from than opioids.[24] Users typically receive little advice and support for discontinuation.[25] Some withdrawal symptoms are identical to the symptoms for which the medication was originally prescribed,[20] and can be acute or protracted in duration. Onset of symptoms from long half-life benzodiazepines might be delayed for up to three weeks, although withdrawal symptoms from short-acting ones often present early, usually within 24–48 hours.[26] There may be no fun-

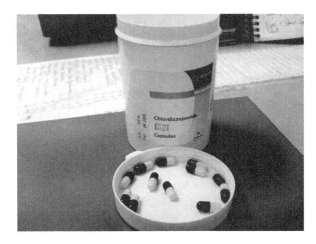

Chlordiazepoxide, 5 mg capsules, are sometimes used as an alternative to diazepam for benzodiazepine withdrawal. Like diazepam, it has a long elimination half-life and long-acting active metabolites.

damental differences in symptoms from either high or low dose discontinuation, but symptoms tend to be more severe from higher doses.[27]

Daytime reemergence and rebound withdrawal symptoms, sometimes called interdose withdrawal, may occur once dependence has set in. Reemergence is the return of symptoms for which the drug was initially prescribed, in contrast, rebound symptoms are a return of the symptoms for which the benzodiazepine was initially taken for, but at a more intense level than before. Withdrawal symptoms, on the other hand, may appear for the first time during dose reduction, and include insomnia, anxiety, distress, weight loss, panic, depression, derealization, and paranoia, and are more commonly associated with short-acting benzodiazepines discontinuation, like triazolam.[21][28] Daytime symptoms can occur after a few days to a few weeks of administration of nightly benzodiazepine use[29][30] or z-drugs such as zopiclone;[31] withdrawal-related insomnia rebounds worse than baseline[32][33] even when benzodiazepines are used intermittently.[34]

The following symptoms may emerge during gradual or abrupt dosage reduction:

- Aches and pains[35]
- Agitation and restlessness[35]
- Akathisia
- Anxiety, possible terror and panic attacks[1][35]
- Blurred vision[35]
- Chest pain[35]
- Depersonalization[36]

- Depression (can be severe),[37] possible suicidal ideation
- Derealisation (feelings of unreality)[38]
- Diarrhea
- Dilated pupils[21]
- Dizziness[35]
- Double vision
- Dry mouth[35]
- Dysphoria[39][40]
- Electric shock sensations[4][41]
- Elevation in blood pressure[42]
- Fatigue and weakness[35]
- Flu-like symptoms[35]
- Gastrointestinal problems [43][43][44]
- Hearing impairment[35]
- Headache[1]
- Hot and cold spells[35]
- Hyperosmia[45]
- Hypertension[46]
- Hypnagogia-hallucinations[16]
- Hypochondriasis[35]
- Increased sensitivity to touch[38]
- Increased sensitivity to sound[35]
- Increased urinary frequency[35]
- Indecision[35]
- Insomnia[47]
- Impaired concentration[1]
- Impaired memory and concentration[35]
- Loss of appetite and weight loss[48]
- Metallic taste[45]
- Mild to moderate Aphasia[45]
- Mood swings[35]
- Muscular spasms, cramps or fasciculations[49]

- Nausea and vomiting[47]
- Nightmares[47]
- Numbness and tingling[35]
- Obsessive compulsive disorder[50][51]
- Paraesthesia[38][45]
- Paranoia[45]
- Perception that stationary objects are moving[38]
- Perspiration[1]
- Photophobia[45]
- Postural hypotension[47]
- REM sleep rebound[52]
- Restless legs syndrome[23]
- Sounds louder than usual[38]
- Stiffness[35]
- Taste and smell disturbances[35]
- Tachycardia[53]
- Tinnitus[54]
- Tremor[55][56]
- Visual disturbances

Rapid discontinuation may result in a more serious syndrome

- Catatonia, which may result in death[57][58][59]
- Confusion[60]
- Convulsions, which may result in death[61][62]
- Coma[63] (rare)
- Delirium tremens[64][65][65]
- Delusions[66]
- Hallucinations
- Hyperthermia[47]
- homicidal ideations[67]
- Mania[68][69]
- Neuroleptic malignant syndrome-like event[70][71] (rare)
- Organic brain syndrome[72]
- Post-traumatic stress disorder[23]
- Psychosis[73][74]
- Suicidal ideation[75]
- Suicide[2][27][76]
- Urges to shout, throw, break things or harm someone[35]
- Violence[77]

As withdrawal progresses, patients often find their physical and mental health improves with improved mood and improved cognition.

2.3.2 Mechanism

Main article: Benzodiazepine dependence § Mechanism
See also: Alcohol withdrawal syndrome § Kindling and Kindling (sedative-hypnotic withdrawal)

The neuroadaptive processes involved in tolerance, dependence, and withdrawal mechanisms implicate both the GABAergic and the glutamatergic systems.[17] Gamma-Aminobutyric acid (GABA) is the major inhibitory neurotransmitter of the central nervous system; roughly one-quarter to one-third of synapses use GABA.[78] GABA mediates the influx of chloride ions through ligand-gated chloride channels called GABAA receptors. When chloride enters the nerve cell, the cell membrane potential hyperpolarizes thereby inhibiting depolarization, or reduction in the firing rate of the post-synaptic nerve cell.[79] Benzodiazepine potentiates the action of GABA,[80] by binding a site between the α and γ subunits of the 5-subunit receptor[81] thereby increasing the frequency of the GABA-gated chloride channel opening in the presence of GABA.[82]

When potentiation is sustained by long-term use, neuroadaptations occur which result in decreased GABAergic response. What is certain is that surface GABAA receptor protein levels are altered in response to benzodiazepine exposure, as is receptor turnover rate.[83] The exact reason for the reduced responsiveness has not been elucidated but down-regulation of the number of receptors has only been observed at some receptor locations including in the pars reticulata of the substantia nigra; down-regulation of the number of receptors or internalization does not appear to be the main mechanism at other locations.[84] Evidence exists for other hypotheses including changes in the receptor conformation, changes in turnover, recycling, or production rates, degree of phosphorylation and receptor gene expression, subunit composition, decreased coupling mechanisms between the GABA and benzodiazepine site, decrease in GABA production, and compensatory increased gutamatergic activity.[17][83] A unified model hypothesis involves a combination of internalization of the receptor, followed by preferential degradation of certain receptor subunits, which provides the nuclear activation for changes in receptor gene transcription.[83]

It has been postulated that when benzodiazepines are cleared from the brain, these neuroadaptations are "unmasked", leading to unopposed excitability of the neuron.[85] Glutamate is the most abundant excitatory neurotransmitter in the vertebrate nervous system.[86] Increased glutamate excitatory activity during withdrawal may lead to sensitization or kindling of the CNS, possibly leading to worsening cognition and symptomatology and making each subsequent withdrawal period worse.[87][88][89] Those who have a prior history of withdrawing from benzodiazepines are found to be less likely to succeed the next time around.[90]

2.3.3 Diagnosis

In severe cases, the withdrawal reaction or protracted withdrawal may exacerbate or resemble serious psychiatric and medical conditions, such as mania, schizophrenia, agitated depression, panic disorder generalised anxiety disorder, and complex partial seizures and, especially at high doses, seizure disorders.[21] Failure to recognize discontinuation symptoms can lead to false evidence for the need to take benzodiazepines, which in turn leads to withdrawal failure and reinstatement of benzodiazepines, often to higher doses. Pre-existing disorder or other causes typically do not improve, where as symptoms of protracted withdrawal gradually improve over the ensuing months.[21] For this reason at least six months should have elapsed after benzodiazepines cessation before re-evaluating the symptoms and updating a diagnosis.

Symptoms may lack a psychological cause and can fluctuate in intensity with periods of good and bad days until eventual recovery.[91][92]

2.3.4 Prevention

According to the British National Formulary, it is better to withdraw too slowly rather than too quickly from benzodiazepines.[26] The rate of dosage reduction is best carried out so as to minimize the symptoms' intensity and severity. Anecdotally, a slow rate of reduction may reduce the risk of developing a severe protracted syndrome.

Long half-life benzodiazepines like diazepam or chlordiazepoxide are preferred to minimize rebound effects, and are available in low potency dose forms. Some people may not fully stabilize between dose reductions, even when the rate of reduction is slowed. Such people sometimes simply need to persist as they may not feel better until they have been fully withdrawn from them for a period of time.[93]

2.3.5 Management

Psychological interventions may provide a small but significant additional benefit over gradual dose reduction alone at post-cessation and at follow-up.[94] The psychological interventions studied were relaxation training, cognitive-behavioral treatment of insomnia, and self-monitoring of consumption and symptoms, goal-setting, management of withdrawal and coping with anxiety.[94]

With sufficient motivation and the proper approach, almost anyone can successfully withdraw from benzodiazepines. However, a prolonged and severe syndrome can lead to collapsed marriages, business failures, bankruptcy, committal to a hospital, and the most serious adverse effect, suicide.[2] As such, long-term users should not be forced to discontinue against their will.[4] Over-rapid withdrawal, lack of explanation, and failure to reassure individuals that they are experiencing temporary withdrawal symptoms led some people to experience increased panic and fears they are going mad, with some people developing a condition similar to post-traumatic stress disorder as a result. A slow withdrawal regimen, coupled with reassurance from family, friends, and peers improves the outcome.[4][16]

Medications and interactions

While some substitutive pharmacotherapies may have promise, current evidence is insufficient to support their use.[94] Some studies found that the abrupt substitution of substitutive pharmacotherapy was actually less effective than gradual dose reduction alone, and only three studies found benefits of adding either melatonin,[95] paroxetine,[96] or trazodone and valproate[97] in conjunction with a gradual dose reduction.[94]

- Antipsychotics are generally ineffective for benzodiazepine withdrawal-related psychosis.[41][98] Antipsychotics should be avoided during benzodiazepine withdrawal as they tend to aggravate withdrawal symptoms, including convulsions.[26][99][100][101] Some antipsychotic agents may be more risky during withdrawal than others, especially clozapine, olanzapine or low potency phenothiazines (e.g., chlorpromazine), as they lower the seizure threshold and can worsen withdrawal effects; if used, extreme caution is required.[102]

- Barbiturates are cross tolerant to benzodiazepines and should be avoided.

- Benzodiazepines or cross tolerant drugs should be avoided after discontinuation, even occasionally. These include the nonbenzodiazepines Z-drugs, which have a similar mechanism of action. This is because tolerance to benzodiazepines has been demonstrated to be still present at four months to two years after withdrawal depending on personal biochemistry. Re-exposures to benzodiazepines typically resulted in a reactivation of the tolerance and benzodiazepine withdrawal syndrome.[103][104]

- Bupropion, which is used primarily as an antidepressant and smoking cessation aid, is contraindicated in persons experiencing abrupt withdrawal from benzodiazepines or other sedative-hypnotics (e.g. alcohol), due to an increased risk of seizures.[105]

- Buspirone augmentation was not found to increase the discontinuation success rate.[6]

- Caffeine may worsen withdrawal symptoms because of its stimulatory properties.[4] Interestingly, at least one animal study has shown some modulation of the benzodiazepine site by caffeine, which produces a lowering of seizure threshold.[106]

- Carbamazepine, an anticonvulsant, appears to have some beneficial effects in the treatment and management of benzodiazepine withdrawal, however, research is limited and thus the ability of experts to make recommendations on its use for benzodiazepine withdrawal is not possible at present.[103]

- Ethanol, the primary alcohol in alcoholic beverages, even mild to moderate use, has been found to be a significant predictor of withdrawal failure, probably because of its cross tolerance with benzodiazepines.[4][103][107]

- Flumazenil has been found to stimulate the reversal of tolerance and the normalization of receptor function. However, further research is needed in the form of randomised trials to demonstrate its role in the treatment of benzodiazepine withdrawal.[108] Flumazenil stimulates the up-regulation and reverses the uncoupling of benzodiazepine receptors to the GABAA receptor, thereby reversing tolerance and reducing withdrawal symptoms and relapse rates.[109][110] Limited research and experience and possible risks involved, the flumazenil detoxification method is controversial and can only be done as an inpatient procedure under medical supervision.

  Flumazenil was found to be more effective than placebo in reducing feelings of hostility and aggression in patients who had been free of benzodiazepines for 4-266 weeks.[111] This may suggest a role for flumazenil in treating protracted benzodiazepine withdrawal symptoms.

  A study into the effects of the benzodiazepine receptor antagonist, flumazenil, on benzodiazepine withdrawal symptoms persisting after withdrawal was carried out by Lader and Morton. Study subjects had been benzodiazepine-free for between one month and five years, but all reported persisting withdrawal effects to varying degrees. Persistent symptoms included clouded thinking, tiredness, muscular symptoms such as neck tension, depersonalisation, cramps and shaking and the characteristic perceptual symptoms of benzodiazepine withdrawal, namely, pins and needles feeling, burning skin, pain and subjective sensations of bodily distortion. Therapy with 0.2–2 mg of flumazenil intravenously was found to decrease these symptoms in a placebo-controlled study. This is of interest as benzodiazepine receptor antagonists are neutral and have no clinical effects. The author of the study suggested the most likely explanation is past benzodiazepine use and subsequent tolerance had locked the conformation of the GABA-BZD receptor complex into an inverse agonist conformation, and the antagonist flumazenil resets benzodiazepine receptors to their original sensitivity. Flumazenil was found in this study to be a successful treatment for protracted benzodiazepine withdrawal syndrome, but further research is required.[112] A study by Professor Borg in Sweden produced similar results in patients suffering from protracted withdrawal.[35] In 2007, Hoffmann–La Roche the makers of flumazenil, acknowledged the existence of protracted benzodiazepine withdrawal syndromes, but did not recommended flumazenil to treat the condition.[113]

- Fluoroquinolone antibiotics[114][115][116] have been noted by Heather Ashton and other authors as increasing the incidence of a CNS toxicity from 1 to 4% in the general population, for benzodiazepine-dependent population or in those undergoing withdrawal from them. This is probably the result of their GABA antagonistic effects as they have been found to competitively displace benzodiazepines from benzodiazepine receptor sites. This antagonism can precipitate acute withdrawal symptoms, that can persist for weeks or months before subsiding. The symptoms include depression, anxiety, psychosis, paranoia, severe insomnia, parathesia, tinnitus, hypersensitivity to light and sound, tremors, status epilepticus, suicidal thoughts and suicide attempt. Fluoroquinolone antibiotics should be contraindicated in patients who are dependent on or in benzodiazepine withdrawal.[4][117][118][119][120] NSAIDs have some mild GABA antagonistic properties and animal research indicate that some may even displace benzodiazepines from their binding site. However, NSAIDs taken in combination with fluoroquinolones cause a very significant increase in GABA antagonism, GABA toxicity, seizures, and other severe adverse effects.[121][122][123]

- Gabapentin can relieve most of the discomfort of benzodiazepine withdrawal; including anxiety, insomnia, irritability, tremor and muscle spasms. However, gabapentin may give rise to its own withdrawal syndrome upon discontinuation if taken continuously for long periods.

- Imidazenil has received some research for management of benzodiazepine withdrawal, but is not currently used in withdrawal.[124]

- Imipramine was found to statistically increase the discontinuation success rate.[6]

- Melatonin augmentation was found to statistically increase the discontinuation success rate for people with insomnia.[6]

- Phenibut may help with the anxiety, insomnia and muscle tension brought on by benzodiazepine discontinuation. However there is a commonly known 'rebound' effect felt with Phenibut that may be exacerbated for people in withdrawal, it is also not recommended to be taken for more than 3 consecutive days to avoid developing a dependency.

- Phenobarbital, (a barbiturate), is used at "detox" or other inpatient facilities to prevent seizures during rapid withdrawal or cold turkey. The phenobarbital is followed by a one- to two-week taper, although a slow taper from phenobarbital is preferred.[21] In a comparison study, a rapid taper using benzodiazepines was found to be superior to a phenobarbital rapid taper.[125][126]

- Pregabalin may help reduce the severity of benzodiazepine withdrawal symptoms,[127] and reduce the risk of relapse.[128]

- Progesterone has been found to be ineffective for managing benzodiazepine withdrawal.[108]

- Propranolol was not found to increase the discontinuation success rate.[6]

- SSRI antidepressants have been found to have little value in the treatment of benzodiazepine withdrawal.[129]

- Tramadol has been found to lower the seizure threshold and should be avoided during benzodiazepine withdrawal.

- Trazodone was not found to increase the discontinuation success rate.[6]

2.3.6 Prognosis

See also: Protracted withdrawal syndrome

The success rate of a minimal intervention where rapid withdrawal is first tried, followed by a systematic tapered discontinuation if the first try was unsuccessful, ranges from 25 to 100% with a median of 58%.[6] Cognitive behavioral therapy was useful to improve success rates for panic disorder, melatonin for insomnia, as was flumazenil and sodium valproate.[6] A ten-year follow-up found that more than half of those who had successfully withdrawn from long-term use were still abstinent two years later, and that if they were able to maintain this state at two years, they were likely to maintain this state at the ten-year followup.[8] One study found that after one year of abstinence from long-term use of benzodiazepines, cognitive, neurological and intellectual impairments had returned to normal.[130]

Those who had a prior psychiatric diagnosis had a similar success rate from a gradual taper at a two-year follow-up.[93][131] Withdrawal from benzodiazepines did not lead to an increased use of antidepressants.[132]

Withdrawal process

It can be too difficult to withdraw from short- or intermediate-acting benzodiazepines because of the intensity of the rebound symptoms felt between doses.[4][133][134][135] Moreover, short-acting benzodiazepines appear to produce a more intense withdrawal syndrome.[136] For this reason, discontinuation is sometimes carried out by first substituting an equivalent dose of a short-acting benzodiazepine to a longer-acting one like diazepam or chlordiazepoxide. Failure to use the correct equivalent amount can precipitate a severe withdrawal reaction.[137] Benzodiazepines with a half-life of more than

24 hours include chlordiazepoxide, diazepam, clobazam, clonazepam, chlorazepinic acid, flurazepam, ketazolam, medazepam, nordazepam, and prazepam. Benzodiazepines with a half-life of less than 24 hours include alprazolam, bromazepam, brotizolam, flunitrazepam, loprazolam, lorazepam, lormetazepam, midazolam, nitrazepam, oxazepam, and temazepam.[8] The resultant equivalent dose is then gradually reduced. The reduction rate used in the Heather Ashton protocol calls for eliminating 10% of the remaining dose every two to four weeks, depending on the severity and response to reductions with the final dose at 0.5 mg dose of diazepam or 5 mg dose of chlordiazepoxide.[4]

Duration

After the last dose has been taken, the acute phase of the withdrawal generally lasts for about two months. Withdrawal symptoms, even from low-dose use, typically persist for six to twelve months and gradually improve over that period,[27][93] however, clinically significant withdrawal symptoms may persist for years, although gradually declining.

A clinical trial of patients taking the benzodiazepine alprazolam for as short as eight weeks triggered protracted symptoms of memory deficits which were still present up to eight weeks after cessation of alprazolam.[138]

Protracted withdrawal syndrome

Protracted withdrawal syndrome refers to symptoms persisting for months or even years. A significant minority of people withdrawing from benzodiazepines, perhaps 10 to 15%, experience a protracted withdrawal syndrome which can sometimes be severe. Symptoms may include tinnitus,[54][139] psychosis, cognitive deficits, gastrointestinal complaints, insomnia, paraesthesia (tingling and numbness), pain (usually in limbs and extremities), muscle pain, weakness, tension, painful tremor, shaking attacks, jerks, and blepharospasm[16] and may occur even without a pre-existing history of these symptoms. Tinnitus occurring during dose reduction or discontinuation of benzodiazepines is alleviated by recommencement of benzodiazepines.

A study testing neuropsychological factors found psychophysiological markers differing from normals, and concluded that protracted withdrawal syndrome was a genuine iatrogenic condition caused by the long-term use.[140] The causes of persisting symptoms are a combination of pharmacological factors such as persisting drug induced receptor changes, psychological factors both caused by the drug and separate from the drug and possibly in some cases, particularly high dose users, structural brain damage or structural neuronal damage.[16][141] Symptoms continue to improve over time, often to the point where people eventually resume their normal lives, even after years of incapacity.[4]

A slow withdrawal rate significantly reduces the risk of a protracted and/or severe withdrawal state. Protracted withdrawal symptoms can be punctuated by periods of good days and bad days. When symptoms increase periodically during protracted withdrawal, physiological changes may be present, including dilated pupils as well as an increase in blood pressure and heart rate.[21] The change in symptoms has been proposed to be due to changes in receptor sensitivity for GABA during the process of tolerance reversal.[4] A meta-analysis found cognitive impairments due to benzodiazepine use show improvements after six months of withdrawal, but the remaining cognitive impairments may be permanent or may require more than six months to reverse.[142]

Protracted symptoms continue to fade over a period of many months or several years. There is no known cure for protracted benzodiazepine withdrawal syndrome except time,[16] however, the medication flumazenil was found to be more effective than placebo in reducing feelings of hostility and aggression in patients who had been free of benzodiazepines for 4–266 weeks.[111] This may suggest a role for flumazenil in treating protracted benzodiazepine withdrawal symptoms.

2.3.7 Epidemiology

The severity and length of the withdrawal syndrome is likely determined by various factors, including rate of tapering, length of use and dosage size, and possible genetic factors.[4][143] Those who have a prior history of withdrawing from benzodiazepines may have a sensitized or kindled central nervous system leading to worsening cognition and symptomatology, and making each subsequent withdrawal period worse.[87][88][89][144]

2.3.8 Special populations

Pediatrics

A neonatal withdrawal syndrome, sometimes severe, can occur when the mother had taken benzodiazepines, especially during the third trimester. Symptoms include hypotonia, apnoeic spells, cyanosis, and impaired metabolic responses to cold stress and seizures. The neonatal benzodiazepine withdrawal syndrome has been reported to persist from hours to months after birth.[145]

A withdrawal syndrome is seen in about 20% of pediatric intensive care unit children after infusions with benzodiazepines or opioids.[146] The likelihood of having the syndrome correlates with total infusion duration and dose, although duration is thought to be more important.[147] Treatment for withdrawal usually involves weaning over an 3 to 21 day period if the infusion lasted for more than a week.[148] Symptoms include tremors, agitation, sleeplessness, inconsolable crying, diarrhea and sweating. In total, over fifty withdrawal symptoms are listed in this review article.[146][149] Environmental measures aimed at easing the symptoms of neonates with severe abstinence syndrome had little impact, but providing a quiet sleep environment helped in mild cases.[146]

Pregnancy

Discontinuing benzodiazepines or antidepressants abruptly due to concerns of teratogenic effects of the medications has a high risk of causing serious complications, so is not recommended. For example, abrupt withdrawal of benzodiazepines or antidepressants has a high risk of causing extreme withdrawal symptoms, including suicidal ideation and a severe rebound effect of the return of the underlying disorder if present. This can lead to hospitalisation and potentially, suicide. One study reported one-third of mothers who suddenly discontinued or very rapidly tapered their medications became acutely suicidal due to 'unbearable symptoms'. One woman had a medical abortion, as she felt she could no longer cope, and another woman used alcohol in a bid to combat the withdrawal symptoms from benzodiazepines. Spontaneous abortions may also result from abrupt withdrawal of psychotropic medications, including benzodiazepines. The study reported physicians generally are not aware of the severe consequences of abrupt withdrawal of psychotropic medications such as benzodiazepines or antidepressants.[75]

The elderly

A study of the elderly who were benzodiazepine dependent found withdrawal could be carried out with few complications and could lead to improvements in sleep and cognitive abilities. At 52 weeks after successful withdrawal, a 22% improvement in cognitive status was found, as well as improved social functioning. Those who remained on benzodiazepines experienced a 5% decline in cognitive abilities, which seemed to be faster than that seen in normal aging, suggesting the longer the intake of benzodiazepines, the worse the cognitive effects become. Some worsening of symptoms were seen in the first few months of benzodiazepine abstinence, but at a 24-week followup, elderly subjects were clearly improved compared to those who remained on benzodiazepines. Improvements in sleep were seen at the 24- and 52-week followups. The authors concluded benzodiazepines were not effective in the long term for sleep problems except in suppressing withdrawal-related rebound insomnia. Improvements were seen between 24 and 52 weeks after withdrawal in many factors, including improved sleep and several cognitive and performance abilities. Some cognitive abilities, which are sensitive to benzodiazepines, as well as age, such as episodic memory did not improve. The authors, however, cited a study in younger patients who at a 3.5-year followup showed no memory impairments and speculated that certain memory functions take longer to recover from chronic benzodiazepine use and further improvements in elderly people's cognitive function may occur beyond 52 weeks after withdrawal. The reason it took 24 weeks for improvements to be seen after cessation of benzodiazepine use was due to the time it takes the brain to adapt to the benzodiazepine-free environment.[150]

At 24 weeks, significant improvements were found, including accuracy of information processing improved, but a decline was seen in those who remained on benzodiazepines. Further improvements were noted at the 52-week followup, indicating ongoing improvements with benzodiazepine abstinence. Younger people on benzodiazepines also experience cognitive deterioration in visual spacial memory, but are not as vulnerable as the elderly to the cognitive effects.[150]

Improved reaction times were noted at 52 weeks in elderly patients free from benzodiazepines. This is an important function in the elderly, especially if they drive a car due to the increased risk of road traffic accidents in benzodiazepine users.[150]

At the 24-week followup, 80% of people had successfully withdrawn from benzodiazepines. Part of the success was attributed to the placebo method used for part of the trial which broke the psychological dependence on benzodiazepines when the elderly patients realised they had completed their gradual reduction several weeks previously, and had only been taking placebo tablets. This helped reassure them they could sleep without their pills.[150]

The authors also warned of the similarities in pharmacology and mechanism of action of the newer nonbenzodiazepine Z drugs.[150]

The elimination half-life of diazepam and chlordiazepoxide, as well as other long half-life benzodiazepines, is twice as long in the elderly compared to younger individuals. Many doctors do not adjust benzodiazepine dosage according to age in elderly patients.[151]

2.3.9 Controversy

Detox facilities may be inappropriate for those who have become tolerant while taking the drug as prescribed, as opposed to recreational use. Such inpatient referrals may be traumatic for non-abusers.[21]

2.3.10 See also

- Alcohol withdrawal syndrome
- Benzodiazepine dependence
- Benzodiazepine equivalence
- Opioid withdrawal syndrome
- Physical dependence
- Post-acute-withdrawal syndrome
- Rebound effect
- SSRI discontinuation syndrome

2.3.11 References

[1] Petursson, H. (1994). "The benzodiazepine withdrawal syndrome". *Addiction* **89** (11): 1455–9. doi:10.1111/j.1360-0443.1994.tb03743.x. PMID 7841856.

[2] Colvin, Rod (26 August 2008). *Overcoming Prescription Drug Addiction: A Guide to Coping and Understanding* (3 ed.). United States of America: Addicus Books. pp. 74–76. ISBN 978-1-886039-88-9. I have treated ten thousand patients for alcohol and drug problems and have detoxed approximately 1,500 patients for benzodiazepines – the detox for the benzodiazepines is one of the hardest detoxes we do. It can take an extremely long time, about half the length of time they have been addicted – the ongoing relentless withdrawals can be so incapacitating it can cause total destruction to one's life – marriages break up, businesses are lost, bankruptcy, hospitalization, and of course suicide is probably the most single serious side effect.

[3] C. Heather Ashton DM. "Chapter III: Benzodiazepine withdrawal symptoms, acute & protracted". Institute of Neuroscience, Newcastle University. Retrieved 29 April 2013. Benzodiazepines : How they work and how to withdraw

[4] Professor Heather Ashton (2002). "Benzodiazepines: How They Work and How to Withdraw".

[5] O'Connor, RD (1993). "Benzodiazepine dependence--a treatment perspective and an advocacy for control". *NIDA research monograph* **131**: 266–9. PMID 8105385.

[6] Voshaar, R. C. O.; Couvée, JE; Van Balkom, AJ; Mulder, PG; Zitman, FG (2006). "Strategies for discontinuing long-term benzodiazepine use: Meta-analysis". *The British Journal of Psychiatry* **189** (3): 213–20. doi:10.1192/bjp.189.3.213. PMID 16946355.

[7] Nutt, David (1986). "Benzodiazepine dependence in the clinic: Reason for anxiety?". *Trends in Pharmacological Sciences* **7**: 457–60. doi:10.1016/0165-6147(86)90420-7.

[8] De Gier, N.; Gorgels, W.; Lucassen, P.; Oude Voshaar, R.; Mulder, J.; Zitman, F. (2010). "Discontinuation of long-term benzodiazepine use: 10-year follow-up". *Family Practice* **28** (3): 253–9. doi:10.1093/fampra/cmq113. PMID 21193495.

[9] Authier, Nicolas; Boucher, Alexandra; Lamaison, Dominique; Llorca, Pierre-Michel; Descotes, Jacques; Eschalier, Alain (2009). "Second Meeting of the French CEIP (Centres d'Évaluation et d'Information sur la Pharmacodépendance). Part II: Benzodiazepine Withdrawal". *Thérapie* **64** (6): 365–70. doi:10.2515/therapie/2009051. PMID 20025839.

[10] Heberlein, A.; Bleich, S.; Kornhuber, J.; Hillemacher, T. (2008). "Benzodiazepin-Abhängigkeit: Ursachen und Behandlungsmöglichkeiten" [Benzodiazepine Dependence: Causalities and Treatment Options]. *Fortschritte der Neurologie · Psychiatrie* (in German) **77** (1): 7–15. doi:10.1055/s-0028-1100831. PMID 19101875.

[11] Lee-chiong, Teofilo (24 April 2008). *Sleep Medicine: Essentials and Review*. Oxford University Press, USA. p. 468. ISBN 0-19-530659-7.

[12] Evans, Katie; Sullivan, Michael J. (2001). "Withdrawal and Medical Issues". *Dual Diagnosis: Counseling the Mentally Ill Substance Abuser* (2nd ed.). Guilford Press. pp. 52–3. ISBN 978-1-57230-446-8.

[13] Lader, M (1987). "Long-term anxiolytic therapy: The issue of drug withdrawal". *The Journal of Clinical Psychiatry*. 48 Suppl: 12–6. PMID 2891684.

[14] Boisse, NR; Periana, RM; Guarino, JJ; Kruger, HS; Samoriski, GM (1986). "Pharmacologic characterization of acute chlordiazepoxide dependence in the rat". *The Journal of Pharmacology and Experimental Therapeutics* **239** (3): 775–83. PMID 3098961.

[15] Boisse, NR; Periana, RM; Guarino, JJ; Kruger, HS (1986). "Acute chlordiazepoxide dependence in the rat: Comparisons to chronic". *NIDA research monograph* **67**: 197–201. PMID 3092067.

[16] Professor Heather Ashton (2004). "Protracted Withdrawal Symptoms From Benzodiazepines". Comprehensive Handbook of Drug & Alcohol Addiction.

[17] Allison, C; Pratt, J.A (2003). "Neuroadaptive processes in GABAergic and glutamatergic systems in benzodiazepine dependence". *Pharmacology & Therapeutics* **98**

(2): 171–95. doi:10.1016/S0163-7258(03)00029-9. PMID 12725868.

[18] Herman, JB; Brotman, AW; Rosenbaum, JF (1987). "Rebound anxiety in panic disorder patients treated with shorter-acting benzodiazepines". *The Journal of Clinical Psychiatry.* 48 Suppl: 22–8. PMID 2889722.

[19] Allgulander, C; Bandelow, B; Hollander, E; Montgomery, SA; Nutt, DJ; Okasha, A; Pollack, MH; Stein, DJ; Swinson, RP; World Council Of, Anxiety (2003). "WCA recommendations for the long-term treatment of generalized anxiety disorder". *CNS spectrums* **8** (8 Suppl 1): 53–61. PMID 14767398.

[20] Salzman, Carl (1993). "Benzodiazepine treatment of panic and agoraphobic symptoms: Use, dependence, toxicity, abuse". *Journal of Psychiatric Research* **27**: 97–110. doi:10.1016/0022-3956(93)90021-S. PMID 7908335.

[21] Gabbard, Glen O. (15 May 2007). *Gabbard's Treatments of Psychiatric Disorders, Fourth Edition (Treatments of Psychiatric Disorders)*. American Psychiatric Publishing. pp. 209–211. ISBN 1-58562-216-8.

[22] Onyett, SR (1989). "The benzodiazepine withdrawal syndrome and its management". *The Journal of the Royal College of General Practitioners* **39** (321): 160–3. PMC 1711840. PMID 2576073.

[23] Ashton, Heather (1991). "Protracted withdrawal syndromes from benzodiazepines". *Journal of Substance Abuse Treatment* **8** (1–2): 19–28. doi:10.1016/0740-5472(91)90023-4. PMID 1675688.

[24] Lindsay, S.J.E.; Powell, Graham E., eds. (28 July 1998). *The Handbook of Clinical Adult Psychology* (2nd ed.). Routledge. p. 363. ISBN 978-0-415-07215-1.

[25] Authier, N.; Balayssac, D.; Sautereau, M.; Zangarelli, A.; Courty, P.; Somogyi, A.A.; Vennat, B.; Llorca, P.-M.; Eschalier, A. (2009). "Benzodiazepine dependence: Focus on withdrawal syndrome". *Annales Pharmaceutiques Françaises* **67** (6): 408–13. doi:10.1016/j.pharma.2009.07.001. PMID 19900604.

[26] Committee on Safety of Medicines (2007). "Hypnotics and anxiolytics". British National Formulary. Retrieved 17 September 2007.(registration required)

[27] Murphy, S. M.; Tyrer, P. (1991). "A double-blind comparison of the effects of gradual withdrawal of lorazepam, diazepam and bromazepam in benzodiazepine dependence". *The British Journal of Psychiatry* **158** (4): 511–6. doi:10.1192/bjp.158.4.511. PMID 1675901.

[28] Adam, Kirstine; Oswald, I. (2008). "Can a Rapidly-eliminated Hypnotic Cause Daytime Anxiety?". *Pharmacopsychiatry* **22** (3): 115–9. doi:10.1055/s-2007-1014592. PMID 2748714.

[29] Scharf, Martin B; Kales, Judith A; Bixler, EO; Jacoby, JA; Schweitzer, PK (1982). "Lorazepam—Efficacy, side effects, and rebound phenomena". *Clinical Pharmacology and Therapeutics* **31** (2): 175–9. doi:10.1038/clpt.1982.27. PMID 6120058.

[30] Walsh, James K; Schweitzer, Paula K; Parwatikar, Sadashiv (1983). "Effects of lorazepam and its withdrawal on sleep, performance, and subjective state". *Clinical Pharmacology and Therapeutics* **34** (4): 496–500. doi:10.1038/clpt.1983.203. PMID 6617072.

[31] Fontaine, Réjean; Beaudry, Paul; Le Morvan, Patrick LE; Beauclair, Linda; Chouinard, GUY (1990). "Zopiclone and Triazolam in Insomnia Associated with Generalized Anxiety Disorder". *International Clinical Psychopharmacology* **5** (3): 173–83. doi:10.1097/00004850-199007000-00002. PMID 2230061.

[32] Kales, Anthony; Bixler, Edward O.; Soldatos, Constantin R.; Jacoby, Judith A.; Kales, Joyce D. (1986). "Lorazepam: Effects on Sleep and Withdrawal Phenomena". *Pharmacology* **32** (3): 121–30. doi:10.1159/000138160. PMID 3960963.

[33] Bonnet, M H; Arand, D L (1999). "The use of lorazepam TID for chronic insomnia". *International Clinical Psychopharmacology* **14** (2): 81–9. doi:10.1097/00004850-199903000-00004. PMID 10220122.

[34] Kales, Anthony; Manfredi, Rocco L; Vgontzas, Alexandras N; Bixler, Edward O; Vela-Bueno, Antonio; Fee, Eric C (1991). "Rebound insomnia after only brief and intermittent use of rapidly eliminated benzodiazepines". *Clinical Pharmacology and Therapeutics* **49** (4): 468–76. doi:10.1038/clpt.1991.55. PMID 2015735.

[35] Saxon, L.; Hjemdahl, P.; Hiltunen, A. J.; Borg, S. (1997). "Effects of flumazenil in the treatment of benzodiazepine withdrawal - a double-blind pilot study". *Psychopharmacology* **131** (2): 153–60. doi:10.1007/s002130050278. PMID 9201803.

[36] Terao, T; Yoshimura, R; Terao, M; Abe, K (1992). "Depersonalization following nitrazepam withdrawal". *Biological Psychiatry* **31** (2): 212–3. doi:10.1016/0006-3223(92)90209-I. PMID 1737083.

[37] Lader, Malcolm (1994). "Anxiety or depression during withdrawal of hypnotic treatments". *Journal of Psychosomatic Research* **38**: 113–23; discussion 118–23. doi:10.1016/0022-3999(94)90142-2. PMID 7799243.

[38] Mintzer, M. Z.; Stoller, K. B.; Griffiths, R. R. (1999). "A controlled study of flumazenil-precipitated withdrawal in chronic low-dose benzodiazepine users". *Psychopharmacology* **147** (2): 200–9. doi:10.1007/s002130051161. PMID 10591888.

[39] Mendelson, WB; Weingartner, H; Greenblatt, DJ; Garnett, D; Gillin, JC (1982). "A clinical study of flurazepam". *Sleep* **5** (4): 350–60. PMID 6761826.

[40] Schöpf, J. (2008). "Withdrawal Phenomena after Long-term Administration of Benzodiazepines a Review of Recent Investigations". *Pharmacopsychiatry* **16** (1): 1–8. doi:10.1055/s-2007-1017439. PMID 6131447.

[41] Shader, RI; Greenblatt, DJ (1981). "The use of benzodiazepines in clinical practice". *British Journal of Clinical Pharmacology*. 11 Suppl 1 (Suppl 1): 5S–9S. doi:10.1111/j.1365-2125.1981.tb01832.x. PMC 1401641. PMID 6133535.

[42] Mintzer, Miriam Z.; Griffiths, Roland R. (2004). "Flumazenil-precipitated withdrawal in healthy volunteers following repeated diazepam exposure". *Psychopharmacology* **178** (2–3): 259–67. doi:10.1007/s00213-004-2009-1. PMID 15452683.

[43] Loeb, P; Adnet, P; Boittiaux, P; Forget, AP; Mille, FX (1997). "Sevrage en benzodiazépines révélé par un syndrome douloureux abdominal pseudochirurgical" [Benzodiazepine withdrawal masquerading as surgical abdominal syndrome]. *Annales Françaises d'Anesthésie et de Réanimation* (in French) **16** (5): 521–2. doi:10.1016/S0750-7658(97)83345-X.

[44] http://www.benzo.org.uk/manual/bzcha03.htm#16[]

[45] Pelissolo, A; Bisserbe, JC (1994). "Dependence on benzodiazepines. Clinical and biological aspects". *L'Encephale* **20** (2): 147–57. PMID 7914165.

[46] Biswas, AK; Feldman, BL; Davis, DH; Zintz, EA (2005). "Myocardial ischemia as a result of severe benzodiazepine and opioid withdrawal". *Clinical toxicology (Philadelphia, Pa.)* **43** (3): 207–9. doi:10.1081/clt-200053099. PMID 15902797.

[47] Bismuth, C; Le Bellec, M; Dally, S; Lagier, G (1980). "Benzodiazepine physical dependence. 6 cases (author's transl)". *La Nouvelle presse medicale* **9** (28): 1941–5. PMID 6106922.

[48] Pecknold, J.C. (1993). "Discontinuation reactions to alprazolam in panic disorder". *Journal of Psychiatric Research* **27**: 155. doi:10.1016/0022-3956(93)90025-W.

[49] Kliniska Färdigheter: Informationsutbytet Mellan Patient Och Läkare, LINDGREN, STEFAN, ISBN 91-44-37271-X (Swedish)

[50] Drummond, Lynne M.; Matthews, Helen P. (1988). "SINGLE CASE STUDY Obsessive-Compulsive Disorder Occurring as a Complication in Benzodiazepine Withdrawal". *The Journal of Nervous and Mental Disease* **176** (11): 688–91. doi:10.1097/00005053-198811000-00008. PMID 3183654.

[51] Matthews, HP; Drummond, LM (1987). "Obsessive-compulsive disorder--a complication of benzodiazepine withdrawal". *The British Journal of Psychiatry* **150**: 272. PMID 3651695.

[52] Pagel, J. F.; Parnes, Bennett L. (2001). "Medications for the Treatment of Sleep Disorders". *The Primary Care Companion to the Journal of Clinical Psychiatry* **3** (3): 118–125. doi:10.4088/PCC.v03n0303. PMC 181172. PMID 15014609.

[53] Van Engelen, BG; Gimbrere, JS; Booy, LH (1993). "Benzodiazepine withdrawal reaction in two children following discontinuation of sedation with midazolam". *The Annals of pharmacotherapy* **27** (5): 579–81. PMID 8347907.

[54] Beeley, L (1991). "Benzodiazepines and tinnitus". *BMJ* **302** (6790): 1465. doi:10.1136/bmj.302.6790.1465.

[55] Mellor, CS; Jain, VK (1982). "Diazepam withdrawal syndrome: Its prolonged and changing nature". *Canadian Medical Association journal* **127** (11): 1093–6. PMC 1862031. PMID 7139456.

[56] Olajide, Dele; Lader, Malcolm (2009). "Depression following withdrawal from long-term benzodiazepine use: A report of four cases". *Psychological Medicine* **14** (4): 937–40. doi:10.1017/S0033291700019899. PMID 6152745.

[57] Rosebush, Patricia I.; Mazurek, Michael F. (1996). "Catatonia After Benzodiazepine Withdrawal". *Journal of Clinical Psychopharmacology* **16** (4): 315–9. doi:10.1097/00004714-199608000-00007. PMID 8835707.

[58] Deuschle, M.F.; Lederbogen, F (2001). "Benzodiazepine Withdrawal - Induced Catatonia". *Pharmacopsychiatry* **34** (1): 41–2. doi:10.1055/s-2001-15188. PMID 11229621.

[59] Kanemoto, Kousuke; Miyamoto, Toshio; Abe, Ryuji (1999). "Ictal catatonia as a manifestation of de novo absence status epilepticus following benzodiazepine withdrawal". *Seizure* **8** (6): 364–6. doi:10.1053/seiz.1999.0309. PMID 10512781.

[60] Uhlenhuth EH; Starcevic V; Qualls C; Antal EJ; Matuzas W; Javaid JI; Barnhill J (October 2006). "Abrupt discontinuation of alprazolam and cognitive style in patients with panic disorder: early effects on mood, performance, and vital signs". *J Clin Psychopharmacol* **26** (5): 519–523. doi:10.1097/01.jcp.0000236653.85791.60. PMID 16974197.

[61] Metten, Pamela; Crabbe, John C (1999). "Genetic Determinants of Severity of Acute Withdrawal from Diazepam in Mice". *Pharmacology Biochemistry and Behavior* **63** (3): 473–9. doi:10.1016/S0091-3057(99)00017-9. PMID 10418790.

[62] Haque, W; Watson, DJ; Bryant, SG (1990). "Death following suspected alprazolam withdrawal seizures: A case report". *Texas medicine* **86** (1): 44–7. PMID 2300914.

[63] De Bard, ML (1979). "Diazepam withdrawal syndrome: A case with psychosis, seizure, and coma". *The American Journal of Psychiatry* **136** (1): 104–5. PMID 103443.

[64] Provini, F.; Cortelli, P.; Montagna, P.; Gambetti, P.; Lugaresi, E. (2008). "Fatal insomnia and agrypnia excitata: Sleep and the limbic system". *Revue Neurologique* **164** (8–9): 692–700. doi:10.1016/j.neurol.2007.11.003. PMID 18805303.

[65] Berezak, A.; Weber, M.; Hansmann, J.; Tulasne, P.A.; Laporte, B.; Ould Ouali, A. (1984). "Dépendance physique aux benzodiazépines dans un contexte traumatologique" [Benzodiazepine physical dependence in traumatology]. *Annales Françaises d'Anesthésie et de Réanimation* (in French) **3** (5): 383–4. doi:10.1016/S0750-7658(84)80078-7.

[66] Keshavan, MS; Moodley, P; Eales, M; Joyce, E; Yeragani, VK (1988). "Delusional depression following benzodiazepine withdrawal". *Canadian Journal of Psychiatry* **33** (7): 626–7. PMID 3197017.

[67] Risse, SC; Whitters, A; Burke, J; Chen, S; Scurfield, RM; Raskind, MA (1990). "Severe withdrawal symptoms after discontinuation of alprazolam in eight patients with combat-induced posttraumatic stress disorder". *The Journal of Clinical Psychiatry* **51** (5): 206–9. PMID 2335496.

[68] Turkington, Douglas; Gill, Paul (1989). "Mania induced by lorazepam withdrawal: A report of two cases". *Journal of Affective Disorders* **17** (1): 93–5. doi:10.1016/0165-0327(89)90028-1. PMID 2525581.

[69] Lapierre, YD; Labelle, A (1987). "Manic-like reaction induced by lorazepam withdrawal". *Canadian Journal of Psychiatry* **32** (8): 697–8. PMID 3690487.

[70] Kawajiri, M; Ohyagi, Y; Furuya, H; Araki, T; Inoue, N; Esaki, S; Yamada, T; Kira, J (2002). "A patient with Parkinson's disease complicated by hypothyroidism who developed malignant syndrome after discontinuation of etizolam". *Rinsho shinkeigaku* **42** (2): 136–9. PMID 12424963.

[71] Strawn, Jeffrey; Keck Jr, PE; Caroff, SN (2007). "Neuroleptic Malignant Syndrome". *American Journal of Psychiatry* **164** (6): 870–6. doi:10.1176/appi.ajp.164.6.870. PMID 17541044.

[72] Khan, A; Joyce, P; Jones, AV (1980). "Benzodiazepine withdrawal syndromes". *The New Zealand medical journal* **92** (665): 94–6. PMID 6107888.

[73] Peh, LH; Mahendran, R (1989). "Psychiatric complications of Erimin abuse". *Singapore medical journal* **30** (1): 72–3. PMID 2595393.

[74] Fruensgaard, K. (1976). "Withdrawal Psychosis: A Study of 30 Consecutive Cases". *Acta Psychiatrica Scandinavica* **53** (2): 105–18. doi:10.1111/j.1600-0447.1976.tb00065.x. PMID 3091.

[75] Einarson, A; Selby, P; Koren, G (2001). "Abrupt discontinuation of psychotropic drugs during pregnancy: Fear of teratogenic risk and impact of counselling". *Journal of Psychiatry & Neuroscience* **26** (1): 44–8. PMC 1408034. PMID 11212593.

[76] Joughin, N.; Tata, P.; Collins, M.; Hooper, C.; Falkowski, J. (1991). "In-patient withdrawal from long-term benzodiazepine use". *Addiction* **86** (4): 449–55. doi:10.1111/j.1360-0443.1991.tb03422.x. PMID 1675899.

[77] Citrome, Leslie; Volavka, Jan (1999). "Violent Patients in the Emergency Setting". *Psychiatric Clinics of North America* **22** (4): 789–801. doi:10.1016/S0193-953X(05)70126-X. PMID 10623971.

[78] Dubuc, Bruno. "Neurotransmitters". The Brain from Top to Bottom. Retrieved 29 April 2013.

[79] Tallman, J F; Gallager, D W (1985). "The Gaba-Ergic System: A Locus of Benzodiazepine Action". *Annual Review of Neuroscience* **8**: 21–44. doi:10.1146/annurev.ne.08.030185.000321. PMID 2858999.

[80] Schoch, P.; Richards, J. G.; Häring, P.; Takacs, B.; Ståhli, C.; Staehelin, T.; Haefely, W.; Möhler, H. (1985). "Co-localization of GABAA receptors and benzodiazepine receptors in the brain shown by monoclonal antibodies". *Nature* **314** (6007): 168–71. Bibcode:1985Natur.314..168S. doi:10.1038/314168a0. PMID 2983231.

[81] Vinkers, Christiaan H.; Olivier, Berend (2012). "Mechanisms Underlying Tolerance after Long-Term Benzodiazepine Use: A Future for Subtype-Selective GABAA Receptor Modulators?". *Advances in Pharmacological Sciences* **2012**: 1. doi:10.1155/2012/416864. PMC 3321276. PMID 22536226.

[82] Study, R. E.; Barker, JL (1981). "Diazepam and (−)-pentobarbital: fluctuation analysis reveals different mechanisms for potentiation of γ-aminobutyric acid responses in cultured central neurons". *Proceedings of the National Academy of Sciences* **78** (11): 7180–4. Bibcode:1981PNAS...78.7180S. doi:10.1073/pnas.78.11.7180. JSTOR 11434. PMC 349220. PMID 6273918.

[83] Bateson, A. (2002). "Basic Pharmacologic Mechanisms Involved in Benzodiazepine Tolerance and Withdrawal". *Current Pharmaceutical Design* **8** (1): 5–21. doi:10.2174/1381612023396681. PMID 11812247.

[84] Tietz, EI; Rosenberg, HC; Chiu, TH (1986). "Autoradiographic localization of benzodiazepine receptor downregulation". *The Journal of Pharmacology and Experimental Therapeutics* **236** (1): 284–92. PMID 3001290.

[85] Koob, G.; Bloom, F. (1988). "Cellular and molecular mechanisms of drug dependence". *Science* **242** (4879): 715–23. Bibcode:1988Sci...242..715K. doi:10.1126/science.2903550. PMID 2903550.

[86] Meldrum, Brian S. (2000). "Glutamate as a Neurotransmitter in the Brain: Review of Physiology and Pathology". *The Journal of Nutrition* **130** (4): 1007S–15S. PMID 10736372.

[87] Stephens, D. N. (1995). "A glutamatergic hypothesis of drug dependence: extrapolations from benzodiazepine receptor ligands". *Behavioural Pharmacology* **6** (5): 425–46. doi:10.1097/00008877-199508000-00004. PMID 11224351.

[88] Dunworth, Sarah J.; Mead, Andy N.; Stephens, David N. (2000). "Previous experience of withdrawal from chronic diazepam ameliorates the aversiveness of precipitated withdrawal and reduces withdrawal-induced c-fos expression in nucleus accumbens". *European Journal of Neuroscience* **12** (4): 1501–8. doi:10.1046/j.1460-9568.2000.00036.x. PMID 10762378.

[89] Rickels, Karl; Schweizer, E; Csanalosi, I; Case, WG; Chung, H (1988). "Long-term Treatment of Anxiety and Risk of Withdrawal: Prospective Comparison of Clorazepate and Buspirone". *Archives of General Psychiatry* **45** (5): 444–50. doi:10.1001/archpsyc.1988.01800290060008. PMID 2895993.

[90] Vorma, Helena; Naukkarinen, Hannu H.; Sarna, Seppo J.; Kuoppasalmi, Kimmo I. (2005). "Predictors of Benzodiazepine Discontinuation in Subjects Manifesting Complicated Dependence". *Substance Use & Misuse* **40** (4): 499–510. doi:10.1081/JA-200052433. PMID 15830732.

[91] Smith, David E.; Wesson, Donald R. (1983). "Benzodiazepine Dependency Syndromes". *Journal of Psychoactive Drugs* **15** (1–2): 85–95. doi:10.1080/02791072.1983.10472127. PMID 6136575.

[92] Landry, MJ; Smith, DE; McDuff, DR; Baughman, OL (1992). "Benzodiazepine dependence and withdrawal: Identification and medical management". *The Journal of the American Board of Family Practice* **5** (2): 167–75. PMID 1575069.

[93] Higgitt, A C; Lader, M H; Fonagy, P (1985). "Clinical management of benzodiazepine dependence". *BMJ* **291** (6497): 688–90. doi:10.1136/bmj.291.6497.688. PMC 1416639. PMID 2864096.

[94] Parr, Jannette M.; Kavanagh, David J.; Cahill, Lareina; Mitchell, Geoffrey; Mcd Young, Ross McD. (2009). "Effectiveness of current treatment approaches for benzodiazepine discontinuation: A meta-analysis". *Addiction* **104** (1): 13–24. doi:10.1111/j.1360-0443.2008.02364.x. PMID 18983627.

[95] Garfinkel, Doron; Zisapel, N; Wainstein, J; Laudon, M (1999). "Facilitation of Benzodiazepine Discontinuation by Melatonin: A New Clinical Approach". *Archives of Internal Medicine* **159** (20): 2456–60. doi:10.1001/archinte.159.20.2456. PMID 10665894.

[96] Nakao, Mutsuhiro; Takeuchi, Takeaki; Nomura, Kyoko; Teramoto, Tamio; Yano, Eiji (2006). "Clinical application of paroxetine for tapering benzodiazepine use in non-major-depressive outpatients visiting an internal medicine clinic". *Psychiatry and Clinical Neurosciences* **60** (5): 605–10. doi:10.1111/j.1440-1819.2006.01565.x. PMID 16958945.

[97] Rickels, K.; Schweizer, E.; Garcia España, F.; Case, G.; Demartinis, N.; Greenblatt, D. (1999). "Trazodone and valproate in patients discontinuing long-term benzodiazepine therapy: Effects on withdrawal symptoms and taper outcome". *Psychopharmacology* **141** (1): 1–5. doi:10.1007/s002130050798. PMID 9952057.

[98] Fruensgaard, K (1977). "Withdrawal psychosis after drugs. Report of a consecutive material". *Ugeskrift for laeger* **139** (29): 1719–22. PMID 898354.

[99] Tagashira, Eijiro; Hiramori, Tameo; Urano, Tomoko; Nakao, Kenzo; Yanaura, Saizo (1981). "Enhancement of drug withdrawal convulsion by combinations of phenobarbital and antipsychotic agents". *The Japanese Journal of Pharmacology* **31** (5): 689–99. doi:10.1254/jjp.31.689. PMID 6118452.

[100] Bobolakis, Ioannis (2000). "Neuroleptic Malignant Syndrome After Antipsychotic Drug Administration During Benzodiazepine Withdrawal". *Journal of Clinical Psychopharmacology* **20** (2): 281–3. doi:10.1097/00004714-200004000-00033. PMID 10770479.

[101] Randall, Michael D; Neil, Karen E (February 2004). "5". *Disease management* (1 ed.). Pharmaceutical Press. p. 62. ISBN 978-0-85369-523-3. Retrieved 1 June 2009.

[102] Ebadi, Manuchair (23 October 2007). "Alphabetical presentation of drugs". *Desk Reference for Clinical Pharmacology* (2nd ed.). USA: CRC Press. p. 512. ISBN 978-1-4200-4743-1.

[103] Lader, Malcolm; Tylee, Andre; Donoghue, John (2009). "Withdrawing Benzodiazepines in Primary Care". *CNS Drugs* **23** (1): 19–34. doi:10.2165/0023210-200923010-00002. PMID 19062773.

[104] Higgitt, A.; Fonagy, P.; Lader, M. (2009). "The natural history of tolerance to the benzodiazepines". *Psychological Medicine. Monograph Supplement* **13**: 1–55. doi:10.1017/S0264180100000412. PMID 2908516.

[105] "Wellbutrin XL Prescribing Information" (PDF). GlaxoSmithKline. December 2008. Archived from the original (PDF) on 2009-03-26. Retrieved 2010-01-16.

[106] Seale, Thomas W.; Carney, John M.; Rennert, Owen M.; Flux, Marinus; Skolnick, Phil (1987). "Coincidence of seizure susceptibility to caffeine and to the benzodiazepine inverse agonist, DMCM, in SWR and CBA inbred mice". *Pharmacology Biochemistry and Behavior* **26** (2): 381–7. doi:10.1016/0091-3057(87)90133-X. PMID 3575358.

[107] Schweizer, Edward; Rickels, K; Case, WG; Greenblatt, DJ (1990). "Long-term Therapeutic Use of Benzodiazepines: II. Effects of Gradual Taper". *Archives of General Psychiatry* **47** (10): 908–15. doi:10.1001/archpsyc.1990.01810220024003. PMID 2222130.

[108] Denis, Cecile; Fatseas, Melina; Lavie, Estelle; Auriacombe, Marc (2006). Denis, Cecile, ed. "Cochrane Database of Systematic Reviews" (3). pp. CD005194. doi:10.1002/14651858.CD005194.pub2. PMID 16856084. |chapter= ignored (help)

[109] Gerra, G.; Zaimovic, A.; Giusti, F.; Moi, G.; Brewer, C. (2002). "Intravenous flumazenil versus oxazepam tapering in the treatment of benzodiazepine withdrawal: A randomized, placebo-controlled study". *Addiction Biology* **7** (4): 385–95. doi:10.1080/1355621021000005973. PMID 14578014.

[110] Little, H.J. (1991). "The benzodiazepines: Anxiolytic and withdrawal effects". *Neuropeptides* **19**: 11–4. doi:10.1016/0143-4179(91)90077-V. PMID 1679209.

[111] L. Saxon, S. Borg & A. J. Hiltunen (August 2010). "Reduction of aggression during benzodiazepine withdrawal: effects of flumazenil". *Pharmacology, biochemistry, and behavior* **96** (2): 148–151. doi:10.1016/j.pbb.2010.04.023. PMID 20451546.

[112] Lader, M. H.; Morton, S. V. (1992). "A pilot study of the effects of flumazenil on symptoms persisting after benzodiazepine withdrawal". *Journal of Psychopharmacology* **6** (3): 357–63. doi:10.1177/026988119200600303. PMID 22291380.

[113] Roche USA (October 2007). "Romazicon" (PDF). Roche Pharmaceuticals USA.

[114] Unseld, E; G Ziegler, A Gemeinhardt, U Janssen, U Klotz (July 1990). "Possible interaction of fluoroquinolones with the benzodiazepine-GABAA-receptor complex (summary)". *Br J Clin Pharmacol* **30** (1): 63–70. Retrieved October 17, 2015.

[115] Ashton, Heather (April 2011). "THE ASHTON MANUAL SUPPLEMENT". *BENZODIAZEPINES: HOW THEY WORK AND HOW TO WITHDRAW*. benzo.org.uk.

[116] Kamath, Ashwin (2013). "Floroquinolone induced neurotoxicity: A review" (PDF). *J. Adv. Pharm. Edu. & Res.* **3** (1): 16–19. Retrieved October 17, 2015.

[117] McConnell, John Girvan (2008). "Benzodiazepine tolerance, dependency, and withdrawal syndromes and interactions with fluoroquinolone antimicrobials". *British Journal of General Practice* **58** (550): 365–6. doi:10.3399/bjgp08X280317. PMC 2435654. PMID 18482496.

[118] Unseld, E; Ziegler, G; Gemeinhardt, A; Janssen, U; Klotz, U (1990). "Possible interaction of fluoroquinolones with the benzodiazepine-GABAA- receptor complex". *British Journal of Clinical Pharmacology* **30** (1): 63–70. doi:10.1111/j.1365-2125.1990.tb03744.x. PMC 1368276. PMID 2167717.

[119] Sternbach, Harvey; State, Rosanne (1997). "Antibiotics: Neuropsychiatric Effects and Psychotropic Interactions". *Harvard Review of Psychiatry* **5** (4): 214–26. doi:10.3109/10673229709000304. PMID 9427014.

[120] Committee on Safety of Medicines; Medicines and Healthcare products Regulatory Agency (2008). "Quinolones". United Kingdom: British National Formulary. Retrieved 16 February 2009. (registration required (help)).

[121] Wong, PT (1993). "Interactions of indomethacin with central GABA systems". *Archives internationales de pharmacodynamie et de therapie* **324**: 5–16. PMID 8297186.

[122] Delanty, Norman (November 2001). "Medication associated seizures". *Seizures: Medical Causes and Management*. Humana Press. pp. 152–153. ISBN 0-89603-827-0.

[123] Green, M. A.; Halliwell, R. F. (1997). "Selective antagonism of the GABAAreceptor by ciprofloxacin and biphenylacetic acid". *British Journal of Pharmacology* **122** (3): 584–90. doi:10.1038/sj.bjp.0701411. PMC 1564969. PMID 9351519.

[124] Auta, J; Costa, E; Davis, J; Guidotti, A (2005). "Imidazenil: An antagonist of the sedative but not the anticonvulsant action of diazepam". *Neuropharmacology* **49** (3): 425–9. doi:10.1016/j.neuropharm.2005.04.005. PMID 15964602.

[125] Sullivan, Mark; Toshima, Michelle; Lynn, Pamela; Roy-Byrne, Peter (1993). "Phenobarbital Versus Clonazepam for Sedative-Hypnotic Taper in Chronic Pain Patients: A Pilot Study". *Annals of Clinical Psychiatry* **5** (2): 123–8. doi:10.3109/10401239309148974. PMID 8348204.

[126] Dr Ray Baker. "Dr Ray Baker's Article on Addiction: Benzodiazepines in Particular". Retrieved 14 February 2009.

[127] Oulis, P.; Konstantakopoulos, G. (2010). "Pregabalin in the treatment of alcohol and benzodiazepines dependence.". *CNS Neurosci Ther* **16** (1): 45–50. doi:10.1111/j.1755-5949.2009.00120.x. PMID 20070788.

[128] Oulis, P.; Konstantakopoulos, G. (Jul 2012). "Efficacy and safety of pregabalin in the treatment of alcohol and benzodiazepine dependence.". *Expert Opin Investig Drugs* **21** (7): 1019–29. doi:10.1517/13543784.2012.685651. PMID 22568872.

[129] Zitman, F. G.; Couvée, JE (2001). "Chronic benzodiazepine use in general practice patients with depression: An evaluation of controlled treatment and taper-off: Report on behalf of the Dutch Chronic Benzodiazepine Working Group". *The British Journal of Psychiatry* **178** (4): 317–24. doi:10.1192/bjp.178.4.317. PMID 11282810.

[130] Tönne, U.; Hiltunen, A. J.; Vikander, B.; Engelbrektsson, K.; Bergman, H.; Bergman, I.; Leifman, H.; Borg, S. (1995). "Neuropsychological changes during steady-state drug use, withdrawal and abstinence in primary benzodiazepine-dependent patients". *Acta Psychiatrica Scandinavica* **91** (5): 299–304. doi:10.1111/j.1600-0447.1995.tb09786.x. PMID 7639085.

[131] Kan, CC; Mickers, FC; Barnhoorn, D (2006). "Short- and long-term results of a systematic benzodiazepine discontinuation programme for psychiatric patients". *Tijdschrift voor psychiatrie* **48** (9): 683–93. PMID 17007474.

[132] Jørgensen, VR (2009). "Benzodiazepine reduction does not imply an increased consumption of antidepressants. A survey of two medical practices". *Ugeskrift for laeger* **171** (41): 2999–3003. PMID 19814928.

[133] Lal R, Gupta S, Rao R, Kattimani S (2007). "Emergency management of substance overdose and withdrawal" (PDF). *Substance Use Disorder* (PDF). World Health Organisation. p. 82. Archived from the original (PDF) on 2010-06-13. Retrieved 2009-06-06. Generally, a longer-acting benzodiazepine such as chlordiazepoxide or diazepam is used and the initial dose titrated downward

[134] Noyes, Russell; Perry, Paul J.; Crowe, Raymond R.; Coryell, William H.; Clancy, John; Yamada, Thoru; Gabel, Janelle (1986). "Seizures Following the Withdrawal of Alprazolam". *The Journal of Nervous and Mental Disease* **174** (1): 50–2. doi:10.1097/00005053-198601000-00009. PMID 2867122.

[135] Noyes Jr, R; Clancy, J; Coryell, WH; Crowe, RR; Chaudhry, DR; Domingo, DV (1985). "A withdrawal syndrome after abrupt discontinuation of alprazolam". *The American Journal of Psychiatry* **142** (1): 114–6. PMID 2857066.

[136] Rickels, Karl; Schweizer, E; Case, WG; Greenblatt, DJ (1990). "Long-term Therapeutic Use of Benzodiazepines: I. Effects of Abrupt Discontinuation". *Archives of General Psychiatry* **47** (10): 899–907. doi:10.1001/archpsyc.1990.01810220015002. PMID 2222129.

[137] Neale, G; Smith, AJ (2007). "Self-harm and suicide associated with benzodiazepine usage". *The British journal of general practice* **57** (538): 407–8. PMC 2047018. PMID 17504594.

[138] Curran, H. V.; Bond, A.; O'Sullivan, G.; Bruce, M.; Marks, I.; Lelliot, P.; Shine, P.; Lader, M. (2009). "Memory functions, alprazolam and exposure therapy: A controlled longitudinal study of agoraphobia with panic disorder". *Psychological Medicine* **24** (4): 969–76. doi:10.1017/S0033291700029056. PMID 7892364.

[139] Busto, Usoa; Fornazzari, Luis; Naranjo, Claudio A. (1988). "Protracted Tinnitus after Discontinuation of Long-Term Therapeutic Use of Benzodiazepines". *Journal of Clinical Psychopharmacology* **8** (5): 359–362. doi:10.1097/00004714-198810000-00010. PMID 2903182.

[140] Higgitt, A.; Fonagy, P.; Toone, B.; Shine, P. (1990). "The prolonged benzodiazepine withdrawal syndrome: Anxiety or hysteria?". *Acta Psychiatrica Scandinavica* **82** (2): 165–8. doi:10.1111/j.1600-0447.1990.tb01375.x. PMID 1978465.

[141] Ashton CH (March 1995). "Protracted Withdrawal From Benzodiazepines: The Post-Withdrawal Syndrome". *Psychiatric Annals* (benzo.org.uk) **25** (3): 174–179.

[142] Barker, M; Greenwood, KM; Jackson, M; Crowe, SF (2004). "Persistence of cognitive effects after withdrawal from long-term benzodiazepine use: A meta-analysis". *Archives of Clinical Neuropsychology* **19** (3): 437–54. doi:10.1016/S0887-6177(03)00096-9. PMID 15033227.

[143] Hood HM, Metten P, Crabbe JC, Buck KJ (February 2006). "Fine mapping of a sedative-hypnotic drug withdrawal locus on mouse chromosome 11". *Genes, Brain and Behavior* **5** (1): 1–10. doi:10.1111/j.1601-183X.2005.00122.x. PMID 16436183.

[144] Vorma, H; Naukkarinen, Hh; Sarna, Sj; Kuoppasalmi, Ki (2005). "Predictors of benzodiazepine discontinuation in subjects manifesting complicated dependence". *Substance Use & Misuse* **40** (4): 499–510. doi:10.1081/JA-200052433. PMID 15830732.

[145] McElhatton, Patricia R. (1994). "The effects of benzodiazepine use during pregnancy and lactation". *Reproductive Toxicology* **8** (6): 461–75. doi:10.1016/0890-6238(94)90029-9. PMID 7881198.

[146] Birchley, Giles (2009). "Opioid and benzodiazepine withdrawal syndromes in the paediatric intensive care unit: A review of recent literature". *Nursing in Critical Care* **14** (1): 26–37. doi:10.1111/j.1478-5153.2008.00311.x. PMID 19154308.

[147] Fontela, Patrícia Scolari; Fontela, Aline; Moraes, Fabrício; Da Silva, Ricardo Bernardi; Sober, Roberta B.; Noer, Francisco; Bruno, Paulo; Einloft, Ana; Garcia, Pedro Celiny Ramos; Piva, Jefferson P. (2003). "Sedation and analgesia in children submitted to mechanical ventilation could be overestimated?". *Jornal de Pediatria* **79** (4): 343–8. doi:10.2223/JPED.1046. PMID 14513134.

[148] Playfor, Stephen; Jenkins, Ian; Boyles, Carolyne; Choonara, Imti; Davies, Gerald; Haywood, Tim; Hinson, Gillian; Mayer, Anton; Morton, Neil; Ralph, Tanya; Wolf, Andrew; United Kingdom Paediatric Intensive Care Society Sedation; Analgesia Neuromuscular Blockade Working Group (2006). "Consensus guidelines on sedation and analgesia in critically ill children". *Intensive Care Medicine* **32** (8): 1125–36. doi:10.1007/s00134-006-0190-x. PMID 16699772.

[149] Ista, Erwin; Van Dijk, Monique; Gamel, Claudia; Tibboel, Dick; De Hoog, Matthijs (2007). "Withdrawal symptoms in children after long-term administration of sedatives and/or analgesics: A literature review. 'Assessment remains troublesome'". *Intensive Care Medicine* **33** (8): 1396–406. doi:10.1007/s00134-007-0696-x. PMID 17541548.

[150] Baillargeon, L; Landreville, P; Verreault, R; Beauchemin, JP; Grégoire, JP; Morin, CM (2003). "Discontinuation of benzodiazepines among older insomniac adults treated with cognitive-behavioural therapy combined with gradual

tapering: A randomized trial". *Canadian Medical Association Journal* **169** (10): 1015–20. PMC 236226. PMID 14609970.

[151] Salzman, Carl (15 May 2004). *Clinical geriatric psychopharmacology* (4th ed.). USA: Lippincott Williams & Wilkins. pp. 450–3. ISBN 978-0-7817-4380-8.

2.3.12 External links

- Benzodiazepine Withdrawal Symptom Relief
- Benzodiazepines: How they work and how to withdraw by Professor Heather Ashton
- The Minor Tranquilliser Project, For support, Camden, UK
- Benzodiazepine withdrawal syndrome at DMOZ

2.4 Benzodiazepine misuse

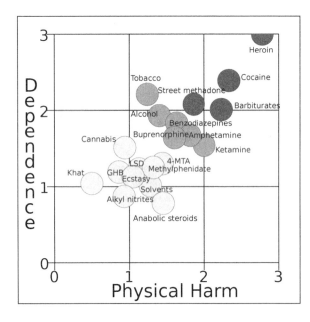

In a poll among medical psychiatrists specialized in addiction treatment, Benzodiazepines were rated as having a similar risk profile as ketamine.[1]

The non-medical use of Benzodiazepine drugs (called **misuse** or **abuse** in public health journals[2]) is the use of benzodiazepines without a prescription, often for recreational purposes, which poses risks of dependence, withdrawal and other long-term effects.[3][4] Benzodiazepines are one of the more common prescription drugs used recreationally. When used recreationally benzodiazepines are usually administered orally but sometimes they are taken intranasally or intravenously. Recreational use produces effects similar to alcohol intoxication.[4][5] In tests in pentobarbital trained rhesus monkeys benzodiazepines produced effects similar to barbiturates.[6] In a 1991 study, triazolam had the highest self-administration rate in cocaine trained baboons, among the five benzodiazepines examined: alprazolam, bromazepam, chlordiazepoxide, lorazepam, triazolam.[7]

A 1985 study found that triazolam and temazepam maintained higher rates of self-injection than a variety of other benzodiazepines.[8]

A 1991 study indicated that diazepam, in particular, had a greater abuse liability among people who were drug abusers than did many of the other benzodiazepines. Some of the available data also suggested that lorazepam and alprazolam are more diazepam-like in having relatively high abuse liability, while oxazepam, halazepam, and possibly chlordiazepoxide, are relatively low in this regard.[9]

A 1991–1993 British study found that the hypnotics flurazepam and temazepam were more toxic than average benzodiazepines in overdose.[10]

A 1995 study found that temazepam is more rapidly absorbed and oxazepam is more slowly absorbed than most other benzodiazepines.[11]

Benzodiazepines have been abused both orally and intravenously. Different benzodiazepines have different abuse potential; the more rapid the increase in the plasma level following ingestion, the greater the intoxicating effect and the more open to abuse the drug becomes. The speed of onset of action of a particular benzodiazepine correlates well with the 'popularity' of that drug for abuse. The two most common reasons for preference were that a benzodiazepine was 'strong' and that it gave a good 'high'.[12]

According to Dr Chris Ford, former clinical director of Substance Misuse Management in General Practice, among drugs of abuse, benzodiazepines are often seen as the 'bad guys' by drug and alcohol workers. Illicit users of benzodiazepines have been found to take higher methadone doses, as well as showing more HIV/HCV risk-taking behaviour, greater poly-drug use, higher levels of psychopathology and social dysfunction. However, there is only limited research into the adverse effects of benzodiazepines in drug misusers and further research is needed to demonstrate whether this is the result of cause or effect.[13]

2.4.1 Background

Benzodiazepines are a commonly abused class of drugs, although there is debate as to whether certain benzodiazepines have higher abuse potential than others.[14] In animal and human studies the abuse potential of benzodiazepines is classed as moderate in comparison to other drugs of abuse.[15] Benzodiazepines are commonly abused by poly drug users, especially heroin addicts, alcoholics or amphetamine addicts when "coming down".[16] but sometimes are misused in isolation as the primary drug of misuse. They can be misused to achieve the high that benzodiazepines produce or more commonly they are used to either enhance the effects of other CNS depressant drugs, to stave off withdrawal effects of other drugs or combat the effects of stimulants. As many as 30–50% of alcoholics are also benzodiazepine misusers.[17] Drug abusers often abuse high doses which makes serious benzodiazepine withdrawal symptoms such as psychosis or convulsions more likely to occur during withdrawal.

Benzodiazepine abuse increases risk taking behaviours such as unprotected sex and sharing of needles amongst intravenous abusers of benzodiazepines. Abuse is also associated with blackouts, memory loss, aggression, violence, and chaotic behaviour associated with paranoia. There is little support for long-term maintenance of benzodiazepine abusers and thus a withdrawal regime is indicated when benzodiazepine abuse becomes a dependence. The main source of illicit benzodiazepines are diverted benzodiazepines obtained originally on prescription; other sources include thefts from pharmacies and pharmaceutical warehouses. Benzodiazepine abuse is steadily increasing and is now a major public health problem. Benzodiazepine abuse is mostly limited to individuals who abuse other drugs, i.e. poly-drug abusers. Most prescribed users do not abuse their medication, however, some high dose prescribed users do become involved with the illicit drug scene. Abuse of benzodiazepines occurs in a wide age range of people and includes teenagers and the old. The abuse potential or drug-liking effects appears to be dose related, with low doses of benzodiazepines having limited drug liking effects but higher doses increasing the abuse potential/drug-liking properties.[18]

2.4.2 Health related complications

See also: Long-term effects of benzodiazepines

Complications of benzodiazepine abuse include drug-related deaths due to overdose especially in combination with other depressant drugs such as opioids. Other complications include: blackouts and memory loss, paranoia, violence and criminal behaviour, risk-taking sexual behaviour, foetal and neonatal risks if taken in pregnancy, dependence, withdrawal seizures and psychosis. Injection of the drug carries risk of: thrombophlebitis, deep vein thrombosis, deep and superficial abscesses, pulmonary microembolism, rhabdomyolysis, tissue necrosis, gangrene requiring amputation, hepatitis B and C, as well as blood borne infections such as HIV infection (caused by sharing injecting equipment).[17] Long-term use of benzodiazepines can worsen pre-existing depression and anxiety and may potentially also cause dementia with impairments in recent and remote memory functions.[19]

Use is widespread among amphetamine users, with those that use amphetamines and benzodiazepines having greater levels of mental health problems and social deterioration. Benzodiazepine injectors are almost four times more likely to inject using a shared needle than non-benzodiazepine-using injectors. It has been concluded in various studies that benzodiazepine use causes greater levels of risk and psycho-social dysfunction among drug misusers.[20] Poly-drug users who also use benzodiazepines appear to engage in more risk taking behavior. Those who use stimulant and depressant drugs are more likely to report adverse reactions from stimulant use, more likely to be injecting stimulants and more likely to have been treated for a drug problem than those using stimulant but not depressant drugs.[21]

2.4.3 Rates of misuse

Little attention has focused on the degree that benzodiazepines are abused as a primary drug of choice, but they are frequently abused alongside other drugs of abuse, especially alcohol, stimulants and opiates.[22] The benzodiazepine most commonly abused can vary from country to country and depends on factors including local popularity as well as which benzodiazepines are available. Nitrazepam for example is commonly abused in Nepal and the United Kingdom,[23][24] whereas in the United States of America where nitrazepam is not available on prescription other benzodiazepines are more commonly abused.[9] In the United Kingdom and Australia there have been epidemics of temazepam abuse. Particular problems with abuse of temazepam are often related to gel capsules being melted and injected and drug-related deaths.[25][26][27] Injecting most benzodiazepines is dangerous because of their relative insolubility in water (with the exception of midazolam), leading to potentially serious adverse health consequences for users.[28][29]

Benzodiazepines are a commonly misused class of drug. A study in Sweden found that benzodiazepines are the most common drug class of forged prescriptions in Sweden.[30] Concentrations of benzodiazepines detected in impaired motor vehicle drivers often exceeding therapeutic doses have been reported in Sweden and in Northern Ireland.[31][32] One of the hallmarks of problematic benzodiazepine drug misuse is escalation of dose. Most licit prescribed users of benzodiazepines do not escalate their dose of benzodiazepines.[33]

2.4.4 Risk factors for misuse

See also: List of benzodiazepines

Individuals with a substance abuse history are at an increased risk of misusing benzodiazepines.[34]

Several (primary research) studies, even into the last decade, claimed, that individuals with a history of familial abuse of alcohol or who are siblings or children of alcoholics appeared to respond differently to benzodiazepines than so called *genetically healthy* persons, with males experiencing increased euphoric effects and females having exaggerated responses to the adverse effects of benzodiazepines.[35][36][37][38]

Whilst all benzodiazepines have abuse potential, certain characteristics increase the potential of particular benzodiazepines for abuse. These characteristics are chiefly practical ones—most especially, availability (often based on popular perception of 'dangerous' versus 'non-dangerous' drugs) through prescribing physicians or illicit distributors. Pharmacological and pharmacokinetic factors are also crucial in determining abuse potentials. A short elimination half-life, high potency and a rapid onset of action are characteristics which increase the abuse potential of benzodiazepines.[39] The following table provides the elimination half-life, relevant potency to other benzodiazepines, speed of onset of action and duration of behavioural effects.[40][41]

*Not all trade names are listed. Click on drug name to see a more comprehensive list.
**The duration of apparent action is usually considerably less than the half-life. With most benzodiazepines, noticeable effects usually wear off within a few hours. Nevertheless, as long as the drug is present it will exert subtle effects within the body. These effects may become apparent during continued use or may appear as withdrawal symptoms when dosage is reduced or the drug is stopped.
***Equivalent doses are based on clinical experience but may vary between individuals.[42]

2.4.5 Drug dependence and withdrawal effects

See also: Benzodiazepine withdrawal syndrome and Benzodiazepine dependence
Sedative hypnotics such as alcohol, benzodiazepines and the barbiturates are notorious for the severe physical dependence that they are capable of inducing which can result in severe withdrawal effects.[43] This severe neuroadaptation is even more profound in high dose drug users and misusers. A high degree of tolerance often occurs in chronic

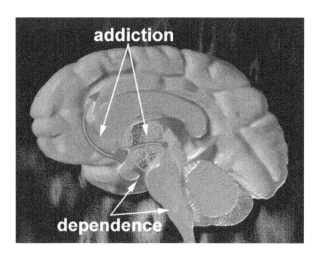

Benzodiazepines can induce a severe benzodiazepine withdrawal syndrome as well as drug seeking behaviour.

benzodiazepine abusers due to the typically high doses they consume which can lead to a severe benzodiazepine dependence. The benzodiazepine withdrawal syndrome seen in chronic high dose benzodiazepine abusers is similar to that seen in therapeutic low dose users but of a more severe nature. Extreme antisocial behaviours in obtaining continued supplies and severe drug-seeking behaviour when withdrawing occurs. The severity of the benzodiazepine withdrawal syndrome has been described by one benzodiazepine drug misuser who stated that[17]

> I'd rather withdraw off heroin any day. If I was withdrawing from benzos you could offer me a gram of heroin or just 20mg of diazepam and I'd take the diazepam every time – I've never been so frightened in my life.

Those who use benzodiazepines intermittently are less likely to develop a dependence and withdrawal symptoms upon dose reduction or cessation of benzodiazepines than those who use benzodiazepines on a daily basis.[17]

Misuse of benzodiazepines is widespread amongst drug misusers; however, many of these people will not require withdrawal management as their use is often restricted to binges or occasional misuse. Benzodiazepine dependence when it occurs requires withdrawal treatment. There is little evidence of benefit from long-term substitution therapy of benzodiazepines, and conversely, there is growing evidence of the harm of long-term use of benzodiazepines, especially higher doses. Therefore, gradual reduction is recommended, titrated against withdrawal symptoms.[44] For withdrawal purposes, stabilisation with a long acting agent such as diazepam is recommended before commencing withdrawal. Chlordiazepoxide (librium), a long-acting benzodiazepine, is gaining attention as an alternative to diazepam in substance abusers dependent on benzodiazepines due to its decreased abuse potential.[22] In individuals dependent on benzodiazepines who have been using benzodiazepines long-term, taper regimes of 6–12 months have been recommended and found to be more successful. More rapid detoxifications e.g. of a month are not recommended as they lead to more severe withdrawal symptoms.[45]

Tolerance leads to a reduction in GABA receptors and function; when benzodiazepines are reduced or stopped this leads to an unmasking of these compensatory changes in the nervous system with the appearance of physical and mental withdrawal effects such as anxiety, insomnia, autonomic hyperactivity and possibly seizures.[39]

Some common withdrawal symptoms which can occur when stopping the use of benzodiazepines include:[17]

All sedative-hypnotics, e.g. alcohol, barbiturates, benzodiazepines and the nonbenzodiazepine Z-drugs have a similar mechanism of action, working on the GABAA receptor complex and are cross tolerant with each other and also have abuse potential. Use of prescription sedative-hypnotics; for example the nonbenzodiazepine Z-drugs often leads to a relapse back into substance misuse with one author stating this occurs in over a quarter of those who have achieved abstinence.[45]

2.4.6 Drug-related crime

See also: Drug-related crime

Problem benzodiazepine use can be associated with various deviant behaviors, including drug-related crime. In a survey of police detainees carried out by the Australian Government, both legal and illegal users of benzodiazepines were found to be more likely to have lived on the streets, less likely to have been in full-time work and more likely to have used heroin or methamphetamines in the past 30 days from the date of taking part in the survey. Benzodiazepine users were also more likely to be receiving illegal incomes and more likely to have been arrested or imprisoned in the previous year. Benzodiazepines were sometimes reported to be used alone, but most often formed part of a poly drug-using problem. Female users were more likely than men to be using heroin, whereas male users were more likely to report amphetamine use. Benzodiazepine users were more likely than non-users to claim government financial benefits and benzodiazepine users who were also poly-drug users were the most likely to be claiming government financial benefits. Those who reported using benzodiazepines alone were found to be in the mid range when compared to other drug using patterns in terms of property crimes and criminal breaches. Of the detainees reporting benzodiazepine use, one in five reported injection use, mostly of illicit temazepam, with some who reported injecting prescribed benzodiazepines. Injection was a concern in this survey due to increased health risks. The main problems highlighted in this survey were concerns of dependence, the potential for overdose of benzodiazepines in combination with opiates and the health problems associated with injection of benzodiazepines.[46]

Benzodiazepines are also sometimes used for drug facilitated sexual assaults and robbery, however, alcohol remains the most common drug involved in drug facilitated assaults. The muscle relaxant, disinhibiting and amnesia producing effects of benzodiazepines are the pharmacological properties which make these drugs effective in drug-facilitated crimes.[47][48] Serial killer Jeffrey Dahmer admitted to using triazolam (Halcion), and occasionally temazepam (Restoril), in order to sedate his victims prior to murdering them.[49]

2.4.7 Drug regulation and enforcement

Europe

Temazepam abuse and seizures have been falling in the UK probably due to its reclassification as Schedule 3 controlled drug with tighter prescribing restrictions and the resultant reduction in availability.[50] A total of 2.75 million temazepam capsules were seized in the Netherlands by authorities between 1996 and 1999.[51] In Northern Ireland statistics of individuals attending drug addiction treatment centers found that benzodiazepines were the 2nd most commonly reported main problem drugs (31 percent of attendees). Cannabis was the top with 35 percent of individuals reporting it as their main problem drug. The statistics showed that treatment for benzodiazepines as the main problematic drug had more than doubled from the previous year and was a growing problem in Northern Ireland.[52]

Oceania

Benzodiazepines are common drugs of abuse in Australia and New Zealand, particularly among those who may also be using other illicit drugs. The intravenous use of temazepam poses the greatest threat to those who misuse benzodiazepines. Simultaneous consumption of temazepam with heroin is a potential risk factor of overdose. An Australian study of non-fatal heroin overdoses, noted that 26% of heroin users had consumed temazepam at the time of their overdose. This is consistent with a NSW investigation of coronial files from 1992. Temazepam was found in 26% of heroin-related deaths. Temazepam, including tablet formulations, are used intravenously. In an

Australian study of 210 heroin users who used temazepam, 48% had injected it. Although abuse of benzodiazepines has decreased over the past few years, temazepam continues to be a major drug of abuse in Australia. In certain states like Victoria and Queensland, temazepam accounts for most benzodiazepine sought by forgery of prescriptions and through pharmacy burglary. Darke, Ross & Hall found that different benzodiazepines have different abuse potential. The more rapid the increase in the plasma level following ingestion, the greater the intoxicating effect and the more open to abuse the drug becomes. The speed of onset of action of a particular benzodiazepine correlates well with the 'popularity' of that drug for abuse. The two most common reasons for preference for a benzodiazepine were that it was the 'strongest' and that it gave a good 'high'.[12]

North America

Abuse of benzodiazepine drugs is a serious problem in North America. The most frequently abused of the benzodiazepines in both the United States and Canada are alprazolam, clonazepam, lorazepam and diazepam.[53]

East and Southeast Asia

Abuse of benzodiazepines is a serious problem throughout East and Southeast Asia.

The Central Narcotics Bureau of Singapore seized 94,200 nimetazepam tablets in 2003. This is the largest nimetazepam seizure recorded since nimetazepam became a controlled drug under the Misuse of Drugs Act in 1992. In Singapore nimetazepam is a Class C controlled drug.[54]

In Hong Kong abuse of prescription medicinal preparations continued in 2006 and seizures of midazolam (120,611 tablets), nimetazepam/nitrazepam (17,457 tablets), triazolam (1,071 tablets), diazepam (48,923 tablets) and chlordiazepoxide (5,853 tablets) were made. Heroin addicts used such tablets (crushed and mixed with heroin) to prolong the effect of the narcotic and ease withdrawal symptoms.[55]

2.4.8 Legal status

In the United States, benzodiazepines are Schedule IV drugs under the Federal Controlled Substances Act, even when not on the market (for example, nitrazepam and bromazepam). Flunitrazepam is subject to more stringent regulations in certain states and temazepam prescriptions require specially coded pads in certain states.

In Canada, possession of benzodiazepines is legal for personal use. All benzodiazepines are categorized as Schedule IV substances under the Controlled Drugs and Substances Act.[56]

In the United Kingdom, the benzodiazepines are schedule 4 controlled drugs, except for flunitrazepam, temazepam and midazolam, which are schedule 3 controlled drugs and carry stronger penalties for possession and trafficking.[57][58]

In the Netherlands, since October 1993, benzodiazepines, including formulations containing less than 20 mg of temazepam, are all placed on List 2 of the Opium Law. A prescription is needed for possession of all benzodiazepines. Temazepam formulations containing 20 mg or greater of the drug are placed on List 1, thus requiring prescriptions to be written in the List 1 format.[59]

In East Asia and Southeast Asia, temazepam and nimetazepam are often heavily controlled and restricted. In certain countries, triazolam, flunitrazepam, flutoprazepam and midazolam are also restricted or controlled to certain degrees. In Hong Kong, all benzodiazepines are regulated under Schedule 1 of Hong Kong's Chapter 134 *Dangerous Drugs Ordinance*.[60] Previously only brotizolam, flunitrazepam and triazolam were classed as dangerous drugs.[61]

Internationally, benzodiazepines are categorized as Schedule IV controlled drugs, apart from flunitrazepam which is a Schedule III drug under the Convention on Psychotropic Substances.[62]

2.4.9 See also

- Drug abuse
- Benzodiazepine overdose
- Effects of long-term benzodiazepine use

2.4.10 References

[1] Nutt, D.; King, L. A.; Saulsbury, W.; Blakemore, C. (2007). "Development of a rational scale to assess the harm of drugs of potential misuse". *The Lancet* **369** (9566): 1047–1053. doi:10.1016/S0140-6736(07)60464-4. PMID 17382831.

[2] "Benzodiazepine dependence: reduce the risk". *NPS MedicineWise*.

[3] Tyrer, P.; Silk, K. R., eds. (2008). "Treatment of Sedative-Hypnotic Dependence". *Cambridge Textbook of Effective Treatments in Psychiatry* (1st ed.). Cambridge University Press. p. 402. ISBN 978-0-521-84228-0.

[4] Griffiths, R. R.; Johnson, M. W. (2005). "Relative Abuse Liability of Hypnotic Drugs: A Conceptual Framework and Algorithm for Differentiating among Compounds" (pdf). *Journal of Clinical Psychiatry* **66** (Suppl 9): 31–41. PMID 16336040.

[5] Sheehan, M. F.; Sheehan, D. V.; Torres, A.; Coppola, A.; Francis, E. (1991). "Snorting Benzodiazepines". *The American Journal of Drug and Alcohol Abuse* **17** (4): 457–468. doi:10.3109/00952999109001605. PMID 1684083.

[6] Woolverton, W. L.; Nader, M. A. (December 1995). "Effects of several benzodiazepines, alone and in combination with flumazenil, in rhesus monkeys trained to discriminate pentobarbital from saline". *Psychopharmacology (Berl.)* **122** (3): 230–236. doi:10.1007/BF02246544. PMID 8748392.

[7] Griffiths, R. R.; Lamb, R. J.; Sannerud, C. A.; Ator, N. A.; Brady, J. V. (1991). "Self-Injection of Barbiturates, Benzodiazepines and other Sedative-Anxiolytics in Baboons". *Psychopharmacology (Berl.)* **103** (2): 154–161. doi:10.1007/BF02244196. PMID 1674158.

[8] GRIFFITHS, Roland R.; RICHARD J. LAMB; NANCY A. ATOR; JOHN D. ROACHE; JOSEPH V. BRADY (1985). "Relative Abuse Liability of Triazolam: Experimental Assessment in Animals and Humans" (PDF). *Neuroscience & Biobehavioral Reviews* **9** (1): 133–151. doi:10.1016/0149-7634(85)90039-9. Retrieved 18 August 2012.

[9] Griffiths, R. R.; Wolf, B. (August 1990). "Relative Abuse Liability of different Benzodiazepines in Drug Abusers". *Journal of Clinical Psychopharmacology* **10** (4): 237–243. doi:10.1097/00004714-199008000-00002. PMID 1981067.

[10] Serfaty, M.; Masterton, G. (September 1993). "Fatal poisonings attributed to benzodiazepines in Britain during the 1980s". *British Journal of Psychiatry* **163** (3): 386–393. doi:10.1192/bjp.163.3.386. PMID 8104653.

[11] Buckley, N. A.; Dawson, A. H.; Whyte, I. M.; O'Connell, D. L. (1995). "Relative toxicity of benzodiazepines in overdose.". *British Medical Journal* **310** (6974): 219–21. doi:10.1136/bmj.310.6974.219. PMC 2548618. PMID 7866122.

[12] Australian Government; Medical Board (2006). "ACT MEDICAL BOARD – STANDARDS STATEMENT – PRESCRIBING OF BENZODIAZEPINES" (pdf). Australia: ACT medical board. Retrieved 13 September 2011.

[13] Chris Ford (2009). "What is possible with benzodiazepines". UK: Exchange Supplies, 2009 National Drug Treatment Conference.

[14] Dart, R. C. (2003). *Medical Toxicology* (3rd ed.). USA: Lippincott Williams & Wilkins. p. 819. ISBN 978-0-7817-2845-4.

[15] Griffiths, R. R.; Weerts, E. M. (November 1997). "Benzodiazepine Self-Administration in Humans and Laboratory Animals – Implications for Problems of Long-Term Use and Abuse". *Psychopharmacology (Berl.)* **134** (1): 1–37. doi:10.1007/s002130050422. PMID 9399364.

[16] Jones, AW; Holmgren A (April 2013). "Amphetamine abuse in Sweden: subject demographics, changes in blood concentrations over time, and the types of coingested substances". *Journal of Clinical Psychopharmacology* **33** (2): 248–252. doi:10.1097/JCP.0b013e3182870310. PMID 23422398. Retrieved 3 November 2013.

[17] Ashton, C. H. (2002). "BENZODIAZEPINE ABUSE". *Drugs and Dependence*. Harwood Academic Publishers. Retrieved 25 September 2007.

[18] Caan, W.; de Belleroche, J., eds. (2002). "Benzodiazepine Abuse". *Drink, Drugs and Dependence: From Science to Clinical Practice* (1st ed.). Routledge. pp. 197–211. ISBN 978-0-415-27891-1.

[19] Galanter, M.; Kleber, H. D. (2008). *The American Psychiatric Publishing Textbook of Substance Abuse Treatment* (4th ed.). United States: American Psychiatric Publishing Inc. p. 197. ISBN 978-1-58562-276-4.

[20] Darke, S.; Ross, J.; Cohen, J. (1994). "The Use of Benzodiazepines among Regular Amphetamine Users". *Addiction* **89** (12): 1683–1690. doi:10.1111/j.1360-0443.1994.tb03769.x. PMID 7866252.

[21] Williamson, S.; Gossop, M.; Powis, B.; Griffiths, P.; Fountain, J.; Strang, J. (1997). "Adverse effects of stimulant drugs in a community sample of drug users". *Drug and Alcohol Dependence* **44** (2–3): 87–94. doi:10.1016/S0376-8716(96)01324-5. PMID 9088780.

[22] Karch, S. B. (2006). *Drug Abuse Handbook* (2nd ed.). USA: CRC Press. p. 572. ISBN 978-0-8493-1690-6.

[23] Chatterjee, A.; Uprety, L.; Chapagain, M.; Kafle, K. (1996). "Drug abuse in Nepal: a rapid assessment study". *Bulletin on Narcotics* **48** (1–2): 11–33. PMID 9839033.

[24] Garretty, D. J.; Wolff, K.; Hay, A. W.; Raistrick, D. (January 1997). "Benzodiazepine misuse by drug addicts". *Annals of Clinical Biochemistry* **34** (Pt 1): 68–73. doi:10.1177/000456329703400110. PMID 9022890.

[25] Wilce, H. (June 2004). "Temazepam capsules: What was the problem?". *Australian Prescriber* **27** (3): 58–59.

[26] Ashton, H. (2002). "Benzodiazepine Abuse". *Drugs and Dependence*. London & New York: Harwood Academic Publishers. Retrieved 2007-11-25.

[27] Hammersley, R.; Cassidy, M. T.; Oliver, J. (1995). "Drugs associated with drug-related deaths in Edinburgh and Glasgow, November 1990 to October 1992". *Addiction* **90** (7): 959–965. doi:10.1046/j.1360-0443.1995.9079598.x. PMID 7663317.

[28] Wang, E.C.; Chew, F. S. (2006). "MR Findings of Alprazolam Injection into the Femoral Artery with Microembolization and Rhabdomyolysis" (pdf). *Radiology Case Reports* **1** (3).

[29] "DB00404 (Alprazolam)". Canada: DrugBank. 26 August 2008.

[30] Bergman, U.; Dahl-Puustinen, M. L. (1989). "Use of prescription forgeries in a drug abuse surveillance network". *European Journal of Clinical Pharmacology* **36** (6): 621–623. doi:10.1007/BF00637747. PMID 2776820.

[31] Jones, A. W.; Holmgren, A.; Kugelberg, F. C. (April 2007). "Concentrations of scheduled prescription drugs in blood of impaired drivers: considerations for interpreting the results". *Therapeutic Drug Monitor* **29** (2): 248–260. doi:10.1097/FTD.0b013e31803d3c04. PMID 17417081.

[32] Cosbey, S. H. (December 1986). "Drugs and the impaired driver in Northern Ireland: an analytical survey". *Forensic Science International* **32** (4): 245–58. doi:10.1016/0379-0738(86)90201-X. PMID 3804143.

[33] Lader, M. H. (1999). "Limitations on the use of benzodiazepines in anxiety and insomnia: are they justified?". *European Neuropsychopharmacology: The Journal of the European College of Neuropsychopharmacology* **9** (Suppl 6): S399–405. doi:10.1016/S0924-977X(99)00051-6. PMID 10622686.

[34] Hoffmann–La Roche. "Mogadon". RxMed. Retrieved 26 May 2009.

[35] Ciraulo, D. A.; Barnhill, J. G.; Greenblatt, D. J.; Shader, R. I.; Ciraulo, A. M.; Tarmey, M. F.; Molloy, M. A.; Foti, M. E. (Sep 1988). "Abuse liability and clinical pharmacokinetics of alprazolam in alcoholic men". *The Journal of Clinical Psychiatry* **49** (9): 333–337. PMID 3417618.

[36] Ciraulo, D. A.; Sarid-Segal, O.; Knapp, C.; Ciraulo, A. M.; Greenblatt, D. J.; Shader, R. I. (Jul 1996). "Liability to alprazolam abuse in daughters of alcoholics". *The American Journal of Psychiatry* **153** (7): 956–958. PMID 8659624.

[37] Evans, S. M.; Levin, F. R.; Fischman, M. W. (Jun 2000). "Increased sensitivity to alprazolam in females with a paternal history of alcoholism". *Psychopharmacology* **150** (2): 150–162. doi:10.1007/s002130000421. PMID 10907668.

[38] Streeter, C. C.; Ciraulo, D. A.; Harris, G. J.; Kaufman, M. J.; Lewis, R. F.; Knapp, C. M.; Ciraulo, A. M.; Maas, L. C.; Ungeheuer, M.; Renshaw, P. F.; Szulewski, S. (May 1998). "Functional magnetic resonance imaging of alprazolam-induced changes in humans with familial alcoholism". *Psychiatry Research* **82** (2): 69–82. doi:10.1016/S0925-4927(98)00009-2. PMID 9754450.

[39] Longo, L. P.; Johnson, B. (April 2000). "Addiction: Part I. Benzodiazepines – Side effects, abuse risk and alternatives". *America Family Physician* **61** (7): 2121–2128. PMID 10779253.

[40] Galanter, M.; Kleber, H. D. (1 July 2008). *The American Psychiatric Publishing Textbook of Substance Abuse Treatment* (4th ed.). United States of America: American Psychiatric Publishing Inc. p. 216. ISBN 978-1-58562-276-4.

[41] Shader, R. I.; Greenblatt, D. J. (1981). "The use of benzodiazepines in clinical practice" (pdf). *British Journal of Clinical Pharmacology* **11** (Suppl 1): 5S–9S. doi:10.1111/j.1365-2125.1981.tb01832.x. PMC 1401641. PMID 6133535.

[42] "benzo.org.uk : Benzodiazepine Equivalence Table". *benzo.org.uk*.

[43] Dr Ray Baker. "Dr Ray Baker's Article on Addiction: Benzodiazepines in Particular". Retrieved 14 February 2009.

[44] National Treatment Agency for Substance Misuse (2007). "Drug misuse and dependence – UK guidelines on clinical management" (PDF). United Kingdom: Department of Health.

[45] Gitlow, S. (2006). *Substance Use Disorders: A Practical Guide* (2nd ed.). USA: Lippincott Williams and Wilkins. pp. 103–121. ISBN 978-0-7817-6998-3.

[46] Loxley, W. (2007). "Benzodiazepine use and harms among police detainees in Australia" (pdf). *Trends & Issues in Crime and Criminal Justice* (Canberra, A.C.T.: Australian Institute of Criminology) (336). ISBN 978-1-921185-39-7. Retrieved 2009-06-10.

[47] Schwartz, R. H.; Milteer, R.; LeBeau, M. A. (Jun 2000). "Drug-facilitated sexual assault ('date rape').". *Southern Medical Journal* **93** (6): 558–61. doi:10.1097/00007611-200093060-00002. PMID 10881768.

[48] Goullé, J. P.; Anger, J. P. (Apr 2004). "Drug-facilitated robbery or sexual assault: problems associated with amnesia". *Therapeutical Drug Monitor* **26** (2): 206–210. doi:10.1097/00007691-200404000-00021. PMID 15228166.

[49] Kottler, Jeffrey (2010). *Duped: Lies and Deception in Psychotherapy*. Routledge. ISBN 978-0-415-87624-7.

[50] The Scottish Government (3 June 2008). "Statistical Bulletin – Drug Seizures by Scottish Police Forces, 2005/2006 and 2006/2007" (pdf). *Crime and Justice Series*. Scotland: scotland.gov.uk. Retrieved 13 February 2009.

[51] INCB (January 1999). "Operation of the international drug control system" (pdf). incb.org. Retrieved 13 February 2009.

[52] Northern Ireland Government (October 2008). "Statistics from the Northern Ireland Drug Misuse Database: 1 April 2007 – 31 March 2008" (pdf). Northern Ireland: Department of Health and Social Services and Public Safety.

[53] United States Government; U.S. Department of Health and Human Services (2006). "Drug Abuse Warning Network, 2006: National Estimates of Drug-Related Emergency Department Visits". Substance Abuse and Mental Health Services Administration. Retrieved 9 February 2009.

[54] Central Narcotics Bureau; Singapore Government (2003). "Drug Situation Report 2003". Singapore: cnb.gov.sg. Retrieved 23 September 2011.

[55] Hong Kong Government. "Suppression of Illicit Trafficking and Manufacturing" (pdf). Hong Kong: nd.gov.hk. Retrieved 13 February 2009.

[56] "Controlled Drugs and Substances Act". Canadian Department of Justice. Retrieved 2009-05-27.

[57] Blackpool NHS Primary Care Trust (1 May 2008). "Medicines Management Update" (PDF). United Kingdom National Health Service. Retrieved 2009-05-27.

[58] "List of Drugs Currently Controlled Under The Misuse of Drugs Legislation" (PDF). *Misuse of Drugs Act UK*. British Government. Retrieved 2009-05-27.

[59] "Opium Law" (PDF). Dutch Government. 29 November 2004. Retrieved 2009-05-27.

[60] Hong Kong Government. "DANGEROUS DRUGS ORDINANCE – SCHEDULE 1". *Hong Kong Ordinances*. Hong Kong: hklii.org.

[61] Lee, K. K.; Chan, T. Y.; Chan, A. W.; Lau, G. S.; Critchley, J. A. (1995). "Use and abuse of benzodiazepines in Hong Kong 1990–93 – The impact of regulatory changes". *Journal of Toxicology. Clinical Toxicology* **33** (6): 597–602. doi:10.3109/15563659509010615. PMID 8523479.

[62] International Narcotics Control Board (August 2003). "List of psychotropic substances under international control" (pdf). incb.org. Retrieved 2008-12-17.

2.5 Effects of long-term benzodiazepine use

The **effects of long-term benzodiazepine use** include drug dependence as well as the possibility of adverse effects on cognitive function, physical health, and mental health.[1] Benzodiazepines are generally effective when used therapeutically in the short-term. Most of the problems associated with benzodiazepines result from their long-term use. There are significant physical, mental and social risks associated with the long-term use of benzodiazepines.[2] However, not all people experience problems associated with the long-term use of benzodiazepines.[3] There is evidence that reduction or withdrawal from benzodiazepines can lead to a reduction in anxiety symptoms,[4][5] although some with panic or anxiety issues may respond solely to benzodiazepine treatment. Due to these increasing physical and mental symptoms from long-term use of benzodiazepines, slowly withdrawing from benzodiazepines is recommended for many long-term users.[6] Not everyone, however, experiences problems with long-term use.[7]

Some of the symptoms that could possibly occur as a result of long-term use of benzodiazepines include emotional clouding,[1] flu-like symptoms,[5] nausea, headaches, dizziness, irritability, lethargy, sleep problems, memory impairment, personality changes, aggression, depression, social deterioration as well as employment difficulties, while others never have any side effects from long term benzodiazepine use. One should never abruptly stop using this medicine and should wean themself down to a lower dose under doctor supervision.[8][9][10] While benzodiazepines are highly effective in the short term, adverse effects in some people associated with long-term use including impaired cognitive abilities, memory problems, mood swings, overdoses when combined with other drugs may make the risk-benefit ratio unfavourable, while others experience no ill effects. In addition, benzodiazepines have reinforcing properties in some individuals and thus are considered to be addictive drugs especially in individuals that have a "drug-seeking" behavior; in addition, a physical dependence can develop after a few weeks or months of use.[11] Many of these adverse effects of long-term use of benzodiazepines begin to show improvements three to six months after withdrawal.[12][13]

Other concerns about the effects of long-term benzodiazepine use, in some, include dose escalation, benzodiazepine abuse, tolerance and benzodiazepine dependence and benzodiazepine withdrawal problems. Both physiological tolerance and dependence can lead to a worsening of the adverse effects of benzodiazepines. Increased risk of death has been associated with long-term use of benzodiazepines in several studies, however, other studies have not found increased mortality. Due to conflicting findings in studies regarding benzodiazepines and increased risks of death including from cancer, further research in long-term use of benzodiazepines and mortality risk has been recommended. Most of the research has been conducted in prescribed users of benzodiazepines; even less is known about the mortality risk of illicit benzodiazepine users.[14] The long-term use of benzodiazepines is controversial and has generated significant controversy within the medical profession. Views on the nature and severity of problems with long-term use of benzodiazepines differ from expert to expert and even from country to country; some experts even question whether there is any problem with the long-term use of benzodiazepines.[15] Political controversy, in particular in the UK, also surrounds the long-term use of benzodiazepines, and was subject to the largest class-action lawsuit in the 1980s and 1990s. There have also been allegations of a cover-up by medical bureaucracies and the government.[16]

2.5.1 Symptoms

Effects of long-term benzodiazepine use may include disinhibition, impaired concentration and memory, depression,[17][18] as well as sexual dysfunction.[6][19] The long-term effects of benzodiazepines may differ from the adverse effects seen after acute administration of benzodiazepines.[20] An analysis of cancer patients found that those who took tranquillisers or sleeping tablets had a substantially poorer quality of life on all measurements conducted, as well as a worse clinical picture of symptomatology. Worsening of symptoms such as fatigue, insomnia, pain, dyspnea and constipation was found when compared against those who did not take tranquillisers or sleeping tablets.[21] Most individuals who successfully discontinue hypnotic therapy after a gradual taper and do not take benzodiazepines for 6 months have less severe sleep and anxiety problems, are less distressed and have a general feeling of improved health at 6 month follow up.[13] The use of benzodiazepines for the treatment of anxiety has been found to lead to a significant increase in healthcare costs due to accidents and other adverse effects associated with the long-term use of benzodiazepines.[22]

Cognitive status

Long-term benzodiazepine use can lead to a generalised impairment of cognition, including sustained attention, verbal learning and memory and psychomotor, visuo-motor and visuo-conceptual abilities.[23][24] These effects on cognition exist, although their impact on patient's daily functioning is, in most (but not all cases), insignificant. Transient changes in the brain have been found using neuroimaging studies, but no brain abnormalities have been found in patients treated long term with benzodiazepines.[25] When benzodiazepine users cease long-term benzodiazepine therapy, their cognitive function improves in the first six months, although deficits may be permanent or take longer than six months to return to baseline.[26][27] In the elderly, long-term benzodiazepine therapy is a risk factor for amplifying cognitive decline,[28] although gradual withdrawal is associated with improved cognitive status.[29] A study of alprazolam found that 8 weeks administration of alprazolam resulted in deficits that were detectable after several weeks but not after 3-5 years.[30]

Effect on sleep

Sleep architecture can be adversely affected by benzodiazepine dependence. Possible adverse effects on sleep include induction or worsening of sleep disordered breathing. Long-term use is associated with increased alpha and beta activity, a decrease in K complexes and delta activity. There is also a decrease in stage 1 NREM, NREM stage 3 and 4 sleep and REM sleep as well as a decrease in REM sleep eye movements.[31]

Mental and physical health

Long-term benzodiazepine use may lead to the creation or exacerbation of physical and mental health conditions, which improve after 6 or more months of abstinence. After a period of about 3 to 6 months of abstinence after completion of a gradual-reduction regimen, marked improvements in mental and physical wellbeing become apparent. For example, one study of hypnotic users gradually withdrawn from their hypnotic medication reported after 6 months of abstinence that they had less severe sleep and anxiety problems, were less distressed, and had a general feeling of improved health. Those having remained on hypnotic medication had no improvements in their insomnia, anxiety, or general health ratings.[13] A study found that individuals having withdrawn from benzodiazepines showed a marked reduction in use of medical and mental health services.[32]

Approximately half of patients attending mental health services for conditions including anxiety disorders such as panic disorder or social phobia may be the result of alcohol or benzodiazepine dependence.[33] Sometimes anxiety disorders pre-existed alcohol or benzodiazepine dependence but the alcohol or benzodiazepine dependence often act to keep the anxiety disorders going and often progressively making them worse.[33] Many people who are addicted to alcohol or prescribed benzodiazepines when it is explained to them they have a choice between ongoing ill mental health or quitting and recovering from their symptoms decide on quitting alcohol and or their benzodiazepines. It was noted that every individual has an individual sensitivity level to alcohol or sedative hypnotic drugs and what one person can tolerate without ill health another will suffer very ill health and that even moderate drinking in sensitive individuals can cause rebound anxiety syndromes and sleep disorders. A person who is suffering the toxic effects of alcohol or benzodiazepines will not benefit from other therapies or medications as they do not address the root cause of the symptoms. Recovery from benzodiazepine dependence tends to take a lot longer than recovery from alcohol but people can regain their previous good health.[33] A review of the literature regarding benzodiazepine hypnotic drugs concluded that these drugs cause an unjustifiable risk to the individual and to public health. The risks include dependence, accidents and other adverse effects. Gradual discontinuation of hypnotics leads to improved health without worsening of sleep.[34]

Daily users of benzodiazepines are also at a higher risk of experiencing psychotic symptomatology such as delusions and hallucinations.[35] A study found that of 42 patients treated with alprazolam, up to a third of long-term users of the benzodiazepine drug alprazolam (Xanax) develop depression.[36] Studies have shown that long-term use of benzodiazepines and the benzodiazepine receptor agonist nonbenzodiazepine Z drugs are associated with causing depression as well as a markedly raised suicide risk and an overall increased mortality risk.[37][38]

A study of 50 patients who attended a benzodiazepine withdrawal clinic found that long-term use of benzodiazepines causes a wide range of psychological and physiological disorders. It was found that, after several years of chronic benzodiazepine use, a large portion of patients developed various mental and physical health problems including agoraphobia, irritable bowel syndrome, paraesthesiae, increasing anxiety, and panic attacks, which were not preexisting. The mental health and physical health symptoms induced by long-term benzodiazepine use gradually improved significantly over a period of a year following completion of a slow withdrawal. Three of the 50 patients had wrongly been given a preliminary diagnosis of multiple sclerosis when the symptoms were actually due to chronic benzodiazepine use. Ten of the patients had taken drug overdoses whilst on benzodiazepines, despite the fact that only two of the patients had any prior history of depressive symptomatology. After withdrawal, no patients took any further overdoses after 1 year post-withdrawal. The cause of the deteriorating mental and physical health in a significant proportion of patients was hypothesised to be caused by increasing tolerance where withdrawal type symptoms emerged, despite the administration of stable prescribed doses.[39] Another theory is that chronic benzodiazepine use causes subtle increasing toxicity, which in turn leads to increasing psychopathology in long-term users of benzodiazepines.[40]

Long-term use of benzodiazepines can induce perceptual disturbances and depersonalisation in some people, even in those taking a stable daily dosage, and it can also become a protracted withdrawal feature of the benzodiazepine withdrawal syndrome.[41]

In addition, chronic use of benzodiazepines is a risk factor for blepharospasm.[42] Drug-induced symptoms that resemble withdrawal-like effects can occur on a set dosage as a result of prolonged use, also documented with barbiturate-like substances, as well as alcohol and benzodiazepines. This demonstrates that the effects from chronic use of benzodiazepine drugs is not unique but occurs with other GABAergic sedative hypnotic drugs, i.e., alcohol and barbiturates.[43]

Immune system

Chronic use of benzodiazepines seemed to cause significant immunological disorders in a study of selected outpatients attending a psychopharmacology department.[44] Diazepam and clonazepam have been found to have long-lasting, but not permanent, immunotoxic effects in the fetus of pregnant rats. However, single very high doses of diazepam have been found to cause lifelong immunosuppression in neonatal rats. No studies have been done to assess the immunotoxic effects of diazepam in humans; however, high prescribed doses of diazepam, in humans, has been found to be a major risk of pneumonia, based on a study of people with tetanus. It has been proposed that diazepam may cause long-lasting changes to the GABAA receptors with resultant long-lasting disturbances to behaviour, endocrine function and immune function[45]

Suicide and self-harm

Because benzodiazepines in general may be associated with increased suicide risk, care should be taken when prescribing especially to at risk patients.[46][47] Depressed adolescents who were taking benzodiazepines were found to have a greatly increased risk of self-harm or suicide, although the sample size was small. The effects of benzodiazepines in individuals under the age of 18 requires further research. Additional caution is required in using benzodiazepines in depressed adolescents.[48] Benzodiazepine dependence often results in an increasingly deteriorating clinical picture, which includes social deterioration leading to comorbid alcoholism and drug abuse. Suicide is a common outcome of chronic benzodiazepine dependence. Benzodiazepine misuse or misuse of other CNS depressants increases the risk of suicide in drug misusers.[49][50] 11% of males and 23% of females with a sedative hypnotic misuse habit commit suicide.[51]

Carcinogenicity

There has been some controversy around the possible link between benzodiazepine use and development of cancer; early cohort studies in the 1980s suggested a possible link, but follow-up case-control studies have found no link between benzodiazepines and cancer. In the second U.S. national cancer study in 1982, the American Cancer Society conducted a survey of over 1.1 million participants. A marked increased risk of cancer was found in the users of sleeping pills, mainly benzodiazepines.[52] There have been 15 epidemiologic studies that have suggested that benzodiazepine or nonbenzodiazepine hypnotic drug use is associated with increased mortality, mainly due to increased cancer deaths in humans. The cancers included cancer of the brain, lung, bowel, breast, and bladder, and other neoplasms. It has been hypothesised that either depressed immune function or the viral infections themselves were the cause of the increased rates of cancer. While initially U.S. Food and Drug Administration reviewers expressed concerns about approving the nonbenzodiazepine Z drugs due to concerns of cancer, ultimately they changed their minds and approved the drugs.[53] A recent case-control study, however, found no link between use of benzodiazepines and cancers of the breast, lung, large bowel, lung, uterine lining, ovaries, testes, thyroid, liver, or Hodgkin's Disease, melanoma, or non-Hodgkin's lymphoma.[54] More specific case-control studies since 2000 have shown no link between benzodiazepine use and breast cancer.[55] One study found an association between self-reported benzodiazepine use and development of ovarian cancer, whereas another study found no relationship.[56][57]

Brain damage evidence

In a study in 1980 in a group of 55 consecutively admitted patients having abused exclusively sedatives or hypnotics, neuropsychological performance was significantly lower and signs of intellectual impairment significantly more often diagnosed than in a matched control group taken from the general population. These results suggested a relationship between abuse of sedatives or hypnotics and cerebral disorder.[58]

A publication has asked in 1981 if lorazepam is more toxic than diazepam.[59]

In a study in 1984, 20 patients having taken long-term benzodiazepines were submitted to brain CT scan examinations. Some scans appeared abnormal. The mean ventricular-brain ratio measured by planimetry was increased over mean values in an age- and sex-matched group of control subjects but was less than that in a group of alcoholics. There was no significant relationship between CT scan appearances and the duration of benzodiazepine therapy. The clinical significance of the findings was unclear.[60]

In 1986, it was presumed that permanent brain damage may result from chronic use of benzodiazepines similar to alcohol-related brain damage.[61]

In 1987, 17 high-dose inpatient abusers of benzodiazepines have anecdotally shown enlarged cerebrospinal fluid spaces with associated brain shrinkage. Brain shrinkage reportedly appeared to be dose dependent with low-dose users having less brain shrinkage than higher-dose users.[62]

However, a CT study in 1987 found no evidence of brain shrinkage in prescribed benzodiazepine users.[63]

In 1989, in a 4- to 6-year follow-up study of 30 inpatient benzodiazepine abusers, Neuropsychological function was found to be permanently affected in some chronic high-dose abusers of benzodiazepines . Brain damage similar to alcoholic brain damage was observed. The CT scan abnormalities showed dilatation of the ventricular system. However, unlike alcoholics, sedative hypnotic abusers showed no evidence of widened cortical sulci. The study concluded that, when cerebral disorder is diagnosed in sedative hypnotic benzodiazepine abusers, it is often permanent.[64]

A CT study in 1993 investigated brain damage in benzodiazepine users and found no overall differences to a healthy control group.[65]

A study in 2000 found that long-term benzodiazepine therapy does not result in brain abnormalities.[66]

Withdrawal from high-dose abuse of nitrazepam anecdotally was alleged in 2001 to have caused severe shock of the whole brain with diffuse slow activity on EEG in one patient after 25 years of abuse. After withdrawal, abnormalities in hypofrontal brain wave patterns persisted beyond the withdrawal syndrome, which suggested to the authors that organic brain damage occurred from chronic high-dose abuse of nitrazepam.[67]

Professor Ashton, a leading expert on benzodiazepines from Newcastle University Institute of Neuroscience, has stated that there is no structural damage from benzodiazepines, and advocates for further research into long-lasting or possibly permanent symptoms of long-term use of benzodiazepines as of 1996.[68] She has stated that she believes that the most likely explanation for lasting symptoms is persisting but slowly resolving functional changes at the GABAA benzodiazepine receptor level. Newer and more detailed brain scanning technologies such as PET scans and MRI scans had as of 2002 to her knowledge never been used to investigate the question of whether benzodiazepines cause functional or structural brain damage.[69]

In 2014 studies have found an association between the use of benzodiazepines and an increased risk of dementia but the exact nature of the relationship is still a matter of debate.[70]

2.5.2 History

Benzodiazepines when introduced in 1961 were widely believed to be safe drugs but as the decades went by increased awareness of adverse effects connected to their long-term use became known. There was initially widespread public approval but this was followed by widespread public disapproval and recommendations for more restrictive medical guidelines followed.[71][72] Concerns regarding the long-term effects of benzodiazepines have been raised since 1980.[73] These concerns are still not fully answered. A review in 2006 of the literature on use of benzodiazepine and nonbenzodiazepine hypnotics concluded that more research is needed to evaluate the long-term effects of hypnotic drugs.[74] The majority of the problems of benzodiazepines are related to their long-term use rather than their short-term use.[75] There is growing evidence of the harm of long-term use of benzodiazepines, especially at higher doses. In 2007 the Department of Health recommended that individuals on long-term benzodiazepines are monitored at least every 3 months and also recommends against long-term substitution therapy in benzodiazepine drug misusers due to a lack of evidence base for effectiveness and due to the risks of long-term use.[76] The long-term effects of benzodiazepines are very similar to the long-term effects of alcohol (apart from organ toxicity) and other sedative-hypnotics. Withdrawal effects and dependence are almost identical. A report in 1987 by the Royal College of Psychiatrists in Great Britain reported that any benefits of long-term use of benzodiazepines are likely to be far outweighed by the risks of long-term use.[77] Despite this benzodiazepines are still widely prescribed. The socioeconomic costs of the continued widespread prescribing of benzodiazepines is high.[78]

Political controversy

The Medical Research Council in 1980 recommended that research be conducted into the effects of long-term use of benzodiazepines[79] A 2009 British Government parliamentary inquiry recommended that research into the long-term effects of benzodiazepines must be carried out.[80] The view of the Department of Health is that they have made every effort to make doctors aware of the problems associated with the long-term use of benzodiazepines,[81] as well as the dangers of benzodiazepine drug addiction.[82]

In 1980, the Medicines and Healthcare products Regulatory Agency's Committee on the Safety of Medicines issued guidance restricting the use of benzodiazepines to short-term use and updated and strengthened these warnings in 1988. When asked by Phil Woolas in 1999 whether the Department of Health had any plans to conduct research into the long-term effects of benzodiazepines, the Department replied, saying they have no plans to do so, as benzodiazepines are already restricted to short-term use and monitored by regulatory bodies.[83] In a House of Commons debate, Phil Woolas has claimed that there has been a cover-up with regard to the problems associated with benzodiazepines because they are of too large of a scale for governments, regulatory bodies, and the pharmaceutical industry to deal with. John Hutton stated in response that the Department of Health take the problems of benzodiazepines extremely seriously and are not sweeping the issue under the carpet.[16] In 2010, the All-Party Parliamentary Group on Involuntary Tranquilliser Addiction filed a complaint with the Equality and Human Rights Commission under the Disability Discrimination Act 1995 against the Department of Health and the Department for Work and Pensions alleging discrimination against people with a benzodiazepine prescription drug dependence as a result of denial of specialised treatment services, exclusion from medical treatment, non-recognition of the protracted benzodiazepine withdrawal syndrome, as well as denial of rehabilitation and back to work schemes. Additionally the APPGITA complaint alleged that there is a "*virtual prohibition*" on the collection of statistical information on benzodiazepines across government departments, whereas with other controlled drugs there are enormous volumes of statistical data. The complaint alleged that the discrimination is deliberate, large scale and that government departments are aware of what they are doing.[84][85]

Declassified Medical Research Council meeting The Medical Research Council (UK) held a closed meeting among top UK medical doctors and representatives from the pharmaceutical industry between the dates of 30 October 1980 and 3 April 1981. The meeting was classified under the Public Records Act 1958 until 2014 but became available in 2005 as a result of the Freedom of Information Act. The meeting was called due to concerns that 10–100,000 people could be dependent; this estimate was later revised by the Chairman Professor Malcolm Lader, of the meeting to approximately half a million members of the British public were suspected of being dependent on therapeutic dose levels of benzodiazepines, about half of those on long-term benzodiazepines. It was reported that benzodiazepines may be the third- or fourth-largest drug problem in the UK (the largest being alcohol and tobacco). The Chairman of the meeting followed up after the meeting with additional information, which was forwarded to the Medical Research Council neuroscience board, raising concerns regarding tests that showed definite cortical atrophy in 2 of 14 individuals tested and borderline abnormality in five others. He felt that, due to the methodology used in assessing the scans, the abnormalities were likely an underestimate, and more refined techniques would be more accurate. Also discussed were findings that tolerance to benzodiazepines can be demonstrated by injecting diazepam into long-term users; in normal subjects, increases in growth hormone occurs, whereas in benzodiazepine-tolerant individuals this effect is blunted. Also raised were findings in animal studies that showed the development of tolerance in the form of a 15 percent reduction in binding capacity of benzodiazepines after seven days administration of high doses of the partial agonist benzodiazepine drug flurazepam and a 50 percent reduction in binding capacity after 30 days of a low dose of diazepam. The Chairman was concerned that papers soon to be published would "*stir the whole matter up*" and wanted to be able to say that the Medical Research Council "*had matters under consideration if questions were asked in parliament*". The Chairman felt that it "*was very important, politically that the MRC should be 'one step ahead'*" and recommended epidemiological studies be funded and carried out by Roche Pharmaceuticals and MRC sponsored research conducted into the biochemical effects of long-term use of benzodiazepines. The meeting aimed to identify issues that were likely to arise, alert the Department of Health to the scale of the problem and identify the pharmacology and nature of benzodiazepine dependence and the volume of benzodiazepines being prescribed. The World Health Organisation was also interested in the problem and it was felt the meeting would demonstrate to the WHO that the MRC was taking the issue seriously. Among the psychological effects of long-term use of benzodiazepines discussed was a reduced ability to cope with stress. The Chairman stated that the "*withdrawal symptoms from valium were much worse than many other drugs including, e.g., heroin*". It was stated that the likelihood of withdrawing from benzodiazepines was "*reduced enormously*" if benzodiazepines were prescribed for longer than four months. It was concluded that benzodiazepines are often prescribed inappropriately, for a wide range of conditions and situations. Dr Mason (DHSS) and Dr Moir (SHHD), felt it important to determine the effectiveness and toxicity of benzodiazepines due to the large numbers of people using benzodiazepines for long periods of time before deciding what regulatory action to take.[79]

Controversy resulted in 2010 when the previously secret files came to light over the fact that the Medical Research Council was warned that benzodiazepines prescribed to millions of patients appeared to cause brain shrinkage similar to alcohol abuse in some patients and failed to carry out larger and more rigorous studies. *The Independent on Sunday* reported allegations that "scores" of the 1.5 million the UK public who use benzodiazepines long-term have symptoms that are consistent with brain damage. It has been described as a 'huge scandal' by Jim Dobbin, and legal experts and MPs have predicted a class action lawsuit. A solicitor said she was aware of the past failed litigation against the drug companies and the relevance the documents had to that court case and said it was strange that the documents were kept 'hidden' by the MRC.[86]

Professor Lader, who chaired the MRC meeting, declined to speculate as to why the MRC declined to support his request to set up a unit to further research benzodiazepines and why they did not set up a special safety committee to look into these concerns. Professor Lader stated that he regrets not being more proactive on pursuing the issue, stating that he did not want to be labeled as the guy who pushed only issues with benzos. Professor Ashton also submitted proposals for grant-funded research using MRI, EEG, and cognitive testing in a ramdomised controlled trial to assess whether benzodiazepines have permanent damage to the brain, but similar to Professor Lader got turned down by the MRC.[86]

The MRC spokesperson said they accept the conclusions of Professor Lader's research and said that they fund only research that meets required quality standards of scientific research, and stated that they were and continue to remain receptive to applications for research in this area. No explanation was reported for why the documents were sealed by the Public Records Act.[86]

Jim Dobbin, who chairs the All-Party Parliamentary Group for Involuntary Tranquilliser Addiction, stated that:[86]

> "Many victims have lasting physical, cognitive and psychological problems even after they have withdrawn. We are seeking legal advice because we believe these documents are the bombshell they have been waiting for. The MRC must justify why there was no proper follow-up to Professor Lader's research, no safety committee, no study, nothing to further explore the results. We are talking about a huge scandal here."

The legal director of Action Against Medical Accidents said urgent research must be carried out and said that, if the results of larger studies confirm professor Lader's research, the government and MRC could be faced with one of the biggest group actions for damages the courts have ever seen given the large number of people potentially affected. People who report enduring symptoms postwithdrawal such as neurological pain, headaches, cognitive impairment, and memory loss have been left in the dark as to whether these symptoms are drug-induced damage or not due to the MRC's inaction, it was reported. Professor Lader reported that the results of his research did not surprise his research group given that it was already known that alcohol could cause permanent brain changes.[86]

Class-action lawsuit Benzodiazepines have a unique history in that they were responsible for the largest-ever class-action lawsuit against drug manufacturers in the United Kingdom, in the 1980s and early 1990s, involving 14,000 patients and 1,800 law firms that alleged the manufacturers knew of the dependence potential but intentionally withheld this information from doctors. At the same time, 117 general practitioners and 50 health authorities were sued by patients to recover damages for the harmful effects of dependence and withdrawal. This led some doctors to require a signed consent form from their patients and to recommend that all patients be adequately warned of the risks of dependence and withdrawal before starting treatment with benzodiazepines.[87] The court case against the drug manufacturers never reached a verdict; legal aid had been withdrawn, leading to the collapse of the trial, and there were allegations that the consultant psychiatrists, the expert witnesses, had a conflict of interest. This litigation led

2.5.3 Special populations

Neonatal effects

Benzodiazepines have been found to cause teratogenic malformations.[89] The literature concerning the safety of benzodiazepines in pregnancy is unclear and controversial. Initial concerns regarding benzodiazepines in pregnancy began with alarming findings in animals but these do not necessarily cross over to humans. Conflicting findings have been found in babies exposed to benzodiazepines.[90] A recent analysis of the Swedish Medical Birth Register found an association with preterm births, low birth weight and a moderate increased risk for congenital malformations. An increase in pylorostenosis or alimentary tract atresia was seen. An increase in orofacial clefts was not demonstrated however and it was concluded that benzodiazepines are not major teratogens.[91]

Neurodevelopmental disorders and clinical symptoms are commonly found in babies exposed to benzodiazepines in utero. Benzodiazepine-exposed babies have a low birth weight but catch up to normal babies at an early age, but smaller head circumferences found in benzo babies persists. Other adverse effects of benzodiazepines taken during pregnancy are deviating neurodevelopmental and clinical symptoms including craniofacial anomalies, delayed development of pincer grasp, deviations in muscle tone and pattern of movements. Motor impairments in the babies are impeded for up to 1 year after birth. Gross motor development impairments take 18 months to return to normal but fine motor function impairments persist.[92] In addition to the smaller head circumference found in benzodiazepine-exposed babies mental retardation, functional deficits, long-lasting behavioural anomalies, and lower intelligence occurs.[93][94]

Benzodiazepines, like many other sedative hypnotic drugs causes apoptotic neuronal cell death. However, benzodiazepines do not cause as severe apoptosis to the developing brain as alcohol does.[95][96][97] The prenatal toxicity of benzodiazepines is most likely due to their effects on neurotransmitter systems, cell membranes and protein synthesis.[98] This however, is complicated in that neuropsychological or neuropsychiatric effects of benzodiazepines, if they occur, may not become apparent until later childhood or even adolescence.[99] A review of the literature found data on long-term follow-up regarding neurobehavioural outcomes is very limited.[100] However, a study was conducted that followed up 550 benzodiazepine-exposed children, which found that, overall, most children developed normally. There was a smaller subset of benzodiazepine-exposed children who were slower to develop, but by four years of age most of this subgroup of children had normalised. There were a small number benzodiazepine-exposed children who had continuing developmental abnormalities at 4-year follow-up, but it was not possible to conclude whether these deficits were the result of benzodiazepines or whether social and environmental factors explained the continuing deficits.[101]

Concerns regarding whether benzodiazepines during pregnancy cause major malformations, in particular cleft palet have been hotly debated in the literature. A meta analysis of the data from cohort studies found no link but meta analysis of case control studies did find a significant increase in major malformations (however, the cohort studies were homogenous and the case control studies were heterogeneous, thus reducing the strength of the case control results). There have also been several reports that suggest that benzodiazepines have the potential to cause a syndrome similar to fetal alcohol syndrome, but this has been disputed by a number of studies. As a result of conflicting findings use of benzodiazepines during pregnancy is controversial. The best available evidence suggests that benzodiazepines are not a major cause of birth defects, i.e. major malformations or cleft lip or cleft palet.[102]

Elderly

Significant toxicity from benzodiazepines can occur in the elderly as a result of long-term use.[103] Benzodiazepines, along with antihypertensives and drugs affecting the cholinergic system are the most common cause of drug-induced dementia affecting over 10 percent of patients attending memory clinics.[104][105] Long-term use of benzodiazepines in the elderly can lead to a pharmacological syndrome with symptoms including drowsiness, ataxia, fatigue, confusion, weakness, dizziness, vertigo, syncope, reversible dementia, depression, impairment of intellect, psychomotor and sexual dysfunction, agitation, auditory and visual hallucinations, paranoid ideation, panic, delirium, depersonalisation, sleepwalking, aggressivity, orthostatic hypotension and insomnia. Depletion of certain neurotransmitters and cortisol levels and alterations in immune function and biological markers can also occur.[106] Elderly individuals who have been long-term users of benzodiazepines have been found to have a higher incidence of post-operative confusion.[107] Benzodiazepines have been associated with increased body sway in the elderly, which can potentially lead to fatal accidents including falls. Discontinuation of benzodiazepines leads to improvement in the balance of the body and also leads to improvements in cognitive functions in the elderly benzodiazepine hypnotic users without worsening of insomnia.[108]

A review of the evidence has found that whilst long-term use of benzodiazepines impairs memory, its association with causing dementia is not clear and requires further research.[109] A more recent study found that benzodiazepines are associated with an increased risk of dementia and it is recommended that benzodiazepines are avoided in the elderly.[110]

2.5.4 See also

- Long-term effects of alcohol
- Benzodiazepine withdrawal syndrome
- Benzodiazepine dependence

2.5.5 References

[1] Ayers, Susan (23 August 2007). Baum, Andrew; McManus, Chris; Newman, Stanton; Wallston, Kenneth; Weinman, John, eds. *Cambridge Handbook of Psychology, Health and Medicine* (2nd ed.). Cambridge University Press. p. 677. ISBN 978-0-521-87997-2.

[2] Ford C, Law F (July 2014). "Guidance for the use and reduction of misuse of benzodiazepines and other hypnotics and anxiolytics in general practice" (PDF). *smmgp.org.uk*.

[3] Hammersley D, Beeley L (1996). "The effects of medication on counselling". In Palmer S, Dainow S, Milner P (eds.). *Counselling: The BACP Counselling Reader* **1**. Sage. pp. 211–4. ISBN 978-0-8039-7477-7.

[4] Galanter, Marc (1 July 2008). *The American Psychiatric Publishing Textbook of Substance Abuse Treatment (American Psychiatric Press Textbook of Substance Abuse Treatment)* (4 ed.). American Psychiatric Publishing, Inc. p. 197. ISBN 978-1-58562-276-4.

[5] Lindsay, S.J.E.; Powell, Graham E., eds. (28 July 1998). *The Handbook of Clinical Adult Psychology* (2nd ed.). Routledge. p. 173. ISBN 978-0-415-07215-1.

[6] Haddad, Peter; Deakin, Bill; Dursun, Serdar, eds. (27 May 2004). "Benzodiazepine dependence". *Adverse Syndromes and Psychiatric Drugs: A clinical guide*. Oxford University Press. pp. 240–252. ISBN 978-0-19-852748-0.

[7] Hammersley D, Beeley L (1996). "The effects of medication on counselling". In Palmer S, Dainow S, Milner P. *Counselling: The BACP Counselling Reader* **1**. Sage. pp. 211–4. ISBN 978-0-8039-7477-7.

[8] Onyett SR (April 1989). "The benzodiazepine withdrawal syndrome and its management". *J R Coll Gen Pract* **39** (321): 160–3. PMC 1711840. PMID 2576073.

[9] National Drug Strategy; National Drug Law Enforcement Research Fund (2007). "Benzodiazepine and pharmaceutical opioid misuse and their relationship to crime - An examination of illicit prescription drug markets in Melbourne, Hobart and Darwin" (PDF). Retrieved 27 December 2008.

[10] Juergens, Sm; Morse, Rm (May 1988). "Alprazolam dependence in seven patients". *The American Journal of Psychiatry* **145** (5): 625–7. doi:10.1176/ajp.145.5.625. ISSN 0002-953X. PMID 3258735.

[11] Denis C, Fatséas M, Lavie E, Auriacombe M (July 2006). Denis, Cecile, ed. "Pharmacological interventions for benzodiazepine mono-dependence management in outpatient settings" (PDF). *Cochrane Database Syst Rev* **3**: CD005194. doi:10.1002/14651858.CD005194.pub2. PMID 16856084.

[12] Rickels K, Lucki I, Schweizer E, García-España F, Case WG (April 1999). "Psychomotor performance of long-term benzodiazepine users before, during, and after benzodiazepine discontinuation". *J Clin Psychopharmacol* **19** (2): 107–13. doi:10.1097/00004714-199904000-00003. PMID 10211911.

[13] Belleville G, Morin CM (March 2008). "Hypnotic discontinuation in chronic insomnia: impact of psychological distress, readiness to change, and self-efficacy". *Health Psychol* **27** (2): 239–48. doi:10.1037/0278-6133.27.2.239. PMID 18377143.

[14] Charlson, F; Degenhardt, L; McLaren, J; Hall, W; Lynskey, M (February 2009). "A systematic review of research examining benzodiazepine-related mortality". *Pharmacoepidemiol Drug Saf* **18** (2): 93–103. doi:10.1002/pds.1694. PMID 19125401.

[15] Uzun, S.; Kozumplik, O.; Jakovljević, M.; Sedić, B. (Mar 2010). "Side effects of treatment with benzodiazepines". *Psychiatr Danub* **22** (1): 90–3. PMID 20305598.

[16] Mr. Phil Woolas; Mr. John Hutton (7 Dec 1999). "Benzodiazepines". England: www.parliament.uk. The story of benzodiazepines is of awesome proportions and has been described as a national scandal. The impact is so large that it is too big for Governments, regulatory authorities, and the pharmaceutical industry to address head on, so the scandal has been swept under the carpet. My reasons for bringing the debate to the Chamber are numerous and reflect the many strands that weave through the issue.

[17] Semple, David; Roger Smyth; Jonathan Burns; Rajan Darjee; Andrew McIntosh (2007) [2005]. "13". *Oxford Handbook of Psychiatry*. United Kingdom: Oxford University Press. p. 540. ISBN 0-19-852783-7.

[18] Collier, Judith; Longmore, Murray (2003). "4". In Scally, Peter. *Oxford Handbook of Clinical Specialties* (6 ed.). Oxford University Press. p. 366. ISBN 978-0-19-852518-9.

[19] Cohen LS, Rosenbaum JF (October 1987). "Clonazepam: new uses and potential problems". *J Clin Psychiatry*. 48 Suppl: 50–6. PMID 2889724.

[20] McLeod DR, Hoehn-Saric R, Labib AS, Greenblatt DJ (April 1988). "Six weeks of diazepam treatment in normal women: effects on psychomotor performance and psychophysiology". *J Clin Psychopharmacol* **8** (2): 83–99. doi:10.1097/00004714-198804000-00002. PMID 3372718.

[21] Paltiel O; Marzec-Boguslawska A; Soskolne V; et al. (December 2004). "Use of tranquilizers and sleeping pills among cancer patients is associated with a poorer quality of life" (PDF). *Qual Life Res* **13** (10): 1699–706. doi:10.1007/s11136-004-8745-1. PMID 15651540.

[22] Berger, A.; Edelsberg, J.; Treglia, M.; Alvir, JM.; Oster, G. (Oct 2012). "Change in healthcare utilization and costs following initiation of benzodiazepine therapy for long-term treatment of generalized anxiety disorder: a retrospective cohort study.". *BMC Psychiatry* **12** (1): 177. doi:10.1186/1471-244X-12-177. PMC 3504522. PMID 23088742.

[23] Barker MJ, Greenwood KM, Jackson M, Crowe SF (2004). "Cognitive effects of long-term benzodiazepine use: a meta-analysis". *CNS Drugs* **18** (1): 37–48. doi:10.2165/00023210-200418010-00004. PMID 14731058.

[24] Golombok S; Moodley P; Lader M (May 1988). "Cognitive impairment in long-term benzodiazepine users". *Psychol Med* **18** (2): 365–74. doi:10.1017/S0033291700007911. PMID 2899898.

[25] Stewart SA (2005). "The effects of benzodiazepines on cognition". *J Clin Psychiatry*. 66 Suppl 2: 9–13. PMID 15762814.

[26] Barker MJ, Greenwood KM, Jackson M, Crowe SF (April 2004). "Persistence of cognitive effects after withdrawal from long-term benzodiazepine use: a meta-analysis". *Arch Clin Neuropsychol* **19** (3): 437–54. doi:10.1016/S0887-6177(03)00096-9. PMID 15033227.

[27] Tata PR; Rollings J; Collins M; Pickering A; Jacobson RR (February 1994). "Lack of cognitive recovery following withdrawal from long-term benzodiazepine use". *Psychol Med* **24** (1): 203–13. doi:10.1017/S0033291700026969. PMID 8208885.

[28] Paterniti S, Dufouil C, Alpérovitch A (June 2002). "Long-term benzodiazepine use and cognitive decline in the elderly: the Epidemiology of Vascular Aging Study". *J Clin Psychopharmacol* **22** (3): 285–93. doi:10.1097/00004714-200206000-00009. PMID 12006899.

[29] Carl Salzman; Janina Fisher; Kenneth Nobel; Randy Glassman; Abbie Wolfson; Margaret Kelley (2004). "Cognitive improvement following benzodiazepine discontinuation in elderly nursing home residents" (PDF). *International Journal of Geriatric Psychiatry* **7** (2): 89–93. doi:10.1002/gps.930070205.

[30] Kiliç C, Curran HV, Noshirvani H, Marks IM, Başoğlu M (January 1999). "Long-term effects of alprazolam on memory: a 3.5 year follow-up of agoraphobia/panic patients". *Psychol Med* **29** (1): 225–31. doi:10.1017/S003329179800734X. PMID 10077311.

[31] Lee-chiong, Teofilo (24 April 2008). *Sleep Medicine: Essentials and Review*. Oxford University Press, USA. p. 105. ISBN 0-19-530659-7.

[32] Burke KC, Meek WJ, Krych R, Nisbet R, Burke JD (February 1995). "Medical services use by patients before and after detoxification from benzodiazepine dependence". *Psychiatr Serv* **46** (2): 157–60. doi:10.1176/ps.46.2.157. PMID 7712252.

[33] primary research citation --> Cohen SI (February 1995). "Alcohol and benzodiazepines generate anxiety, panic and phobias". *J R Soc Med* **88** (2): 73–7. PMC 1295099. PMID 7769598.

[34] <Please add first missing authors to populate metadata.> (December 2004). "What's wrong with prescribing hypnotics?". *Drug Ther Bull* **42** (12): 89–93. doi:10.1136/dtb.2004.421289. PMID 15587763.

[35] Tien AY; Anthony JC (August 1990). "Epidemiological analysis of alcohol and drug use as risk factors for psychotic experiences". *J Nerv Ment Dis* **178** (8): 473–80. doi:10.1097/00005053-199017880-00001. PMID 2380692.

[36] Lydiard, Rb; Laraia, Mt; Ballenger, Jc; Howell, Ef (May 1987). "Emergence of depressive symptoms in patients receiving alprazolam for panic disorder". *The American Journal of Psychiatry* **144** (5): 664–5. doi:10.1176/ajp.144.5.664. ISSN 0002-953X. PMID 3578580.

[37] Nathan RG; Robinson D; Cherek DR; Davison S; Sebastian S; Hack M (1 January 1985). "Long-term benzodiazepine use and depression". *Am J Psychiatry* (American Journal of Psychiatry) **142** (1): 144–5. PMID 2857068.

[38] Kripke DF (August 21, 2007). "Greater incidence of depression with hypnotic use than with placebo". *BMC Psychiatry* (pubmed) **7**: 42. doi:10.1186/1471-244X-7-42. PMC 1994947. PMID 17711589.

[39] Professor C Heather Ashton (1987). "Benzodiazepine Withdrawal: Outcome in 50 Patients". *British Journal of Addiction* **82**: 655–671.

[40] Michelini S; Cassano GB; Frare F; Perugi G (July 1996). "Long-term use of benzodiazepines: tolerance, dependence and clinical problems in anxiety and mood disorders". *Pharmacopsychiatry* **29** (4): 127–34. doi:10.1055/s-2007-979558. PMID 8858711.

[41] Ashton H (1991). "Protracted withdrawal syndromes from benzodiazepines". *J Subst Abuse Treat* (benzo.org.uk) **8** (1–2): 19–28. doi:10.1016/0740-5472(91)90023-4. PMID 1675688.

[42] Wakakura M, Tsubouchi T, Inouye J (March 2004). "Etizolam and benzodiazepine induced blepharospasm". *J. Neurol. Neurosurg. Psychiatr.* **75** (3): 506–a. doi:10.1136/jnnp.2003.019869. PMC 1738986. PMID 14966178.

[43] Cookson JC (September 1995). "Rebound exacerbation of anxiety during prolonged tranquilizer ingestion". *J R Soc Med* **88** (9): 544. PMC 1295346. PMID 7562864.

[44] Lechin F; van der Dijs B, Vitelli-Flores G, Báez S, Lechin ME, Lechin AE, Orozco B, Rada I, León G, Jiménez V (February 1994). "Peripheral blood immunological parameters in long-term benzodiazepine users". *Clin Neuropharmacol* **17** (1): 63–72. doi:10.1097/00002826-199402000-00007. PMID 7908607.

[45] Luebke, RW.; Chen, DH.; Dietert, R.; Yang, Y.; King, M.; Luster, MI.; Immunotoxicology, Workgroup (2006). "The comparative immunotoxicity of five selected compounds following developmental or adult exposure". *J Toxicol Environ Health B Crit Rev* **9** (1): 1–26. doi:10.1080/15287390500194326. PMID 16393867.

[46] Neutel CI, Patten SB (November 1997). "Risk of suicide attempts after benzodiazepine and/or antidepressant use". *Ann Epidemiol* **7** (8): 568–74. doi:10.1016/S1047-2797(97)00126-9. PMID 9408553.

[47] Taiminen TJ (January 1993). "Effect of psychopharmacotherapy on suicide risk in psychiatric inpatients". *Acta Psychiatr Scand* **87** (1): 45–7. doi:10.1111/j.1600-0447.1993.tb03328.x. PMID 8093823.

[48] Brent DA; Emslie GJ; Clarke GN; et al. (April 2009). "Predictors of spontaneous and systematically assessed suicidal adverse events in the treatment of SSRI-resistant depression in adolescents (TORDIA) study". *Am J Psychiatry* **166** (4): 418–26. doi:10.1176/appi.ajp.2008.08070976. PMC 3593721. PMID 19223438.

[49] Allgulander C, Borg S, Vikander B (December 1984). "A 4-6-year follow-up of 50 patients with primary dependence on sedative and hypnotic drugs". *Am J Psychiatry* **141** (12): 1580–2. doi:10.1176/ajp.141.12.1580. PMID 6507663.

[50] Wines JD, Saitz R, Horton NJ, Lloyd-Travaglini C, Samet JH (December 2004). "Suicidal behavior, drug use and depressive symptoms after detoxification: a 2-year prospective study". *Drug Alcohol Depend* **76** (Suppl): S21–9. doi:10.1016/j.drugalcdep.2004.08.004. PMID 15555813.

[51] Allgulander C, Ljungberg L, Fisher LD (May 1987). "Long-term prognosis in addiction on sedative and hypnotic drugs analyzed with the Cox regression model". *Acta Psychiatr Scand* **75** (5): 521–31. doi:10.1111/j.1600-0447.1987.tb02828.x. PMID 3604738.

[52] Daniel F. Kripke. "Mortality Associated with Prescription Hypnotics". USA: National Center for Biotechnology Information.

[53] Kripke, Daniel F (2008). "Evidence That New Hypnotics Cause Cancer" (PDF). *Department of Psychiatry, UCSD* (University of California). the likelihood of cancer causation is sufficiently strong now that physicians and patients should be warned that hypnotics possibly place patients at higher risk for cancer.

[54] Rosenberg L; Palmer JR; Zauber AG; et al. (June 1995). "Relation of benzodiazepine use to the risk of selected cancers: breast, large bowel, malignant melanoma, lung, endometrium, ovary, non-Hodgkin's lymphoma, testis, Hodgkin's disease, thyroid, and liver". *Am. J. Epidemiol.* **141** (12): 1153–60. PMID 7771453.

[55] Halapy E, Kreiger N, Cotterchio M, Sloan M (August 2006). "Benzodiazepines and risk for breast cancer". *Ann Epidemiol* **16** (8): 632–6. doi:10.1016/j.annepidem.2005.11.004. PMID 16406246.

[56] Harlow BL; Cramer DW (March 1995). "Self-reported use of antidepressants or benzodiazepine tranquilizers and risk of epithelial ovarian cancer: evidence from two combined case-control studies (Massachusetts, United States)". *Cancer Causes Control* **6** (2): 130–4. doi:10.1007/BF00052773. PMID 7749052.

[57] Dublin S, Rossing MA, Heckbert SR, Goff BA, Weiss NS (February 2002). "Risk of epithelial ovarian cancer in relation to use of antidepressants, benzodiazepines, and other centrally acting medications" (PDF). *Cancer Causes Control* **13** (1): 35–45. doi:10.1023/A:1013969611593. PMID 11899116.

[58] Borg S; Bergman H; Holm L. (1 February 1980). "Neuropsychological impairment and exclusive abuse of sedatives or hypnotics". *The American journal of psychiatry.* **137** (2): 215–7. doi:10.1176/ajp.137.2.215. PMID 7352578.

[59] van Hiele LJ (January 1981). "[Can lorazepam be distinguished from other short-acting benzodiazepines in regard to brain damage and withdrawal symptoms?]". *Ned Tijdschr Geneeskd* (in Dutch and Flemish) **125** (4): 156. PMID 6111030.

[60] Lader, Mh; Ron, M; Petursson, H (Feb 1984). "Computed axial brain tomography in long-term benzodiazepine users". *Psychological Medicine* **14** (1): 203–6. doi:10.1017/S0033291700003214. ISSN 0033-2917. PMID 6143338.

[61] Lennane, Kj (May 1986). "Treatment of benzodiazepine dependence". *The Medical journal of Australia* **144** (11): 594–7. ISSN 0025-729X. PMID 2872582.

[62] Schmauss, C; Krieg, Jc (Nov 1987). "Enlargement of cerebrospinal fluid spaces in long-term benzodiazepine abusers". *Psychological Medicine* **17** (4): 869–73. doi:10.1017/S0033291700000660. ISSN 0033-2917. PMID 2893406.

[63] Perera, Km; Powell, T; Jenner, Fa (Aug 1987). "Computerized axial tomographic studies following long-term use of benzodiazepines". *Psychological Medicine* **17** (3): 775–7. doi:10.1017/S0033291700026003. ISSN 0033-2917. PMID 2888147.

[64] Borg S; Bergman H; Engelbrektson K; Vikander B. (1989). "Dependence on sedative-hypnotics: neuropsychological impairment, field dependence and clinical course in a 5-year follow-up study". *British journal of addiction.* **84** (5): 547–53. doi:10.1111/j.1360-0443.1989.tb00612.x. PMID 2743035.

[65] Moodley, P; Golombok, S; Shine, P; Lader, M (Aug 1993). "Computed axial brain tomograms in long-term benzodiazepine users". *Psychiatry Research* **48** (2): 135–44. doi:10.1016/0165-1781(93)90037-H. PMID 8105500.

[66] Busto, Ue; Bremner, Ke; Knight, K; Terbrugge, K; Sellers, Em (Feb 2000). "Long-term benzodiazepine therapy does not result in brain abnormalities". *Journal of Clinical Psychopharmacology* **20** (1): 2–6. doi:10.1097/00004714-200002000-00002. PMID 10653201.

[67] Kitabayashi Y; Ueda H; Narumoto J; et al. (2001). "Chronic high-dose nitrazepam dependence 123I-IMP SPECT and EEG studies". *Addict Biol* **6** (3): 257–261. doi:10.1080/13556210120056507. PMID 11900604.

[68] Professor C Heather Ashton. "Long-Term Effects of Benzodiazepine Usage: Research Proposals, 1995-96". University of Newcastle - School of Neurosciences: benzo.org.uk. Retrieved 10 December 2008.

[69] Professor C Heather Ashton (29 August 2002). "NO EVIDENCE THAT BENZODIAZEPINES ARE "LOCKED UP" IN TISSUES FOR YEARS". benzo.org.uk. Retrieved 10 December 2008.

[70] Lawrence, Janna (27 September 2014). "Benzodiazepine use is associated with Alzheimer's disease, study finds". *The Pharmaceutical Journal* **293** (7829). Retrieved 2014-10-10.

[71] Marshall, KP.; Georgievskava, Z.; Georgievsky, I. (Jun 2009). "Social reactions to Valium and Prozac: a cultural lag perspective of drug diffusion and adoption". *Res Social Adm Pharm* **5** (2): 94–107. doi:10.1016/j.sapharm.2008.06.005. PMID 19524858.

[72] Fraser AD (October 1998). "Use and abuse of the benzodiazepines". *Ther Drug Monit* **20** (5): 481–9. doi:10.1097/00007691-199810000-00007. PMID 9780123.

[73] Edwards RA, Medlicott RW (November 1980). "Advantages and disadvantages of benzodiazepine prescription". *N. Z. Med. J.* **92** (671): 357–9. PMID 6109269.

[74] Bain KT (June 2006). "Management of chronic insomnia in elderly persons". *Am J Geriatr Pharmacother* **4** (2): 168–92. doi:10.1016/j.amjopharm.2006.06.006. PMID 16860264.

[75] Ashton H (1994). "Guidelines for the rational use of benzodiazepines. When and what to use". *Drugs* **48** (1): 25–40. doi:10.2165/00003495-199448010-00004. PMID 7525193. Retrieved 18 June 2009.

[76] National Treatment Agency for Substance Misuse (2007). "Drug misuse and dependence - UK guidelines on clinical management" (PDF). United Kingdom: Department of Health.

[77] Gitlow, Stuart (1 October 2006). *Substance Use Disorders: A Practical Guide* (2nd ed.). USA: Lippincott Williams and Wilkins. pp. 101–103. ISBN 978-0-7817-6998-3.

[78] Authier, N.; Balayssac, D.; Sautereau, M.; Zangarelli, A.; Courty, P.; Somogyi, AA.; Vennat, B.; Llorca, PM.; Eschalier, A. (November 2009). "Benzodiazepine dependence: focus on withdrawal syndrome". *Ann Pharm Fr* **67** (6): 408–13. doi:10.1016/j.pharma.2009.07.001. PMID 19900604.

[79] Professor Lader; Professor Morgan, Professor Shepherd, Dr Paul Williams, Dr Skegg, Professor Parish, Dr Peter Tyrer, Dr Inman, Dr John Marks (Ex-Roche), Peter Harris (Roche), Tom Hurry (Wyeth). "Benzodiazepine Dependence Medical Research Council headquarters, Closed until 2014 - Opened 2005" (PDF). England: The National Archives. 30 October 1980 - 3 April 1981

[80] DrugScope; Gemma Reay; Dr Brian Iddon MP. "All-Party Parliamentary Drugs Misuse Group - An Inquiry into Physical Dependence and Addiction to Prescription and Over-the-Counter Medication" (PDF). UK: DrugScope.org.uk. Retrieved 21 January 2009. 2007–2008

[81] Dawn Primarolo; David Mellor (18 July 1989). "Benzodiazepines". United Kingdom: Hansard, UK Parliament.

[82] Audrey Wise; Alan Milburn (6 May 1998). "Benzodiazepines". United Kingdom: Handsard, UK Parliament.

[83] Yvette Cooper; Phil Woolas (11 November 1999). "Benzodiazepine". United Kingdom: Handsard, UK Parliament.

[84] Michael Behan; Jim Dobbin (20 July 2009). "ALL-PARTY PARLIAMENTARY GROUP ON INVOLUNTARY TRANQUILLISER ADDICTION, SUBMISSION TO EQUALITIES AND HUMAN RIGHTS COMMISSION" (PDF). AddictionToday.org. The discrimination is large scale, long-standing and deliberate. Government Departments are aware that they are discriminating but reject the available solutions. The discrimination has disastrous effects on the lives of those affected.

[85] Jo Waters (23 March 2010). "Agony of the very unlikely addicts: Thousands of over-60s are hooked on tranquillisers that have turned them into virtual zombies". United Kingdom: Daily Mail.

[86] Nina Lakhani (7 November 2010). "Drugs linked to brain damage 30 years ago". United Kingdom: The Independent on Sunday.

[87] King MB (1992). "Is there still a role for benzodiazepines in general practice?". *Br J Gen Pract* **42** (358): 202–5. PMC 1372025. PMID 1389432.

[88] Peart R (1999-06-01). "Memorandum by Dr Reg Peart". *Minutes of Evidence*. Select Committee on Health, House of Commons, UK Parliament. Retrieved 27 May 2009.

[89] Mazaira S (2005). "[Effects of psychiatric drugs on the fetus and newborn children. Consequences of the treatment of psychiatric disorders during pregnancy and lactation]". *Vertex* (in Spanish) **16** (59): 35–42. PMID 15785787.

[90] McGrath C, Buist A, Norman TR (February 1999). "Treatment of anxiety during pregnancy: effects of psychotropic drug treatment on the developing fetus". *Drug Saf* **20** (2): 171–86. doi:10.2165/00002018-199920020-00006. PMID 10082073.

[91] Wikner BN, Stiller CO, Bergman U, Asker C, Källén B (November 2007). "Use of benzodiazepines and benzodiazepine receptor agonists during pregnancy: neonatal outcome and congenital malformations". *Pharmacoepidemiol Drug Saf* **16** (11): 1203–10. doi:10.1002/pds.1457. PMID 17894421.

[92] L, Laegreid; Hagberg G; Lundberg A (April 1992). "Neurodevelopment in late infancy after prenatal exposure to benzodiazepines—a prospective study". *Neuropediatrics* **23** (2): 60–7. doi:10.1055/s-2008-1071314. PMID 1351263.

[93] L, Laegreid (1990). "Clinical observations in children after prenatal benzodiazepine exposure". *Dev Pharmacol Ther* **15** (3–4): 186–8. PMID 1983095.

[94] Karkos, J (December 1991). "The neurotoxicity of benzodiazepines". *Fortschritte der Neurologie-Psychiatrie* **59** (12): 498–520. doi:10.1055/s-2007-1000726. PMID 1685467.

[95] Ikonomidou C; Bittigau P; Koch C; et al. (August 2001). "Neurotransmitters and apoptosis in the developing brain". *Biochem. Pharmacol.* **62** (4): 401–5. doi:10.1016/S0006-2952(01)00696-7. PMID 11448448.

[96] Gressens P, Mesples B, Sahir N, Marret S, Sola A (April 2001). "Environmental factors and disturbances of brain development". *Semin Neonatol* **6** (2): 185–94. doi:10.1053/siny.2001.0048. PMID 11483023.

[97] Farber NB, Olney JW (December 2003). "Drugs of abuse that cause developing neurons to commit suicide". *Brain Res. Dev. Brain Res.* **147** (1–2): 37–45. doi:10.1016/j.devbrainres.2003.09.009. PMID 14741749.

[98] Karkos J (December 1991). "[The neurotoxicity of benzodiazepines]". *Fortschr Neurol Psychiatr* (in German) **59** (12): 498–520. doi:10.1055/s-2007-1000726. PMID 1685467.

[99] Kellogg CK (1985). "Drugs and chemicals that act on the central nervous system: interpretation of experimental evidence". *Prog. Clin. Biol. Res.* **163C**: 147–53. PMID 3887421.

[100] Austin MP, Mitchell PB (October 1998). "Psychotropic medications in pregnant women: treatment dilemmas". *Med. J. Aust.* **169** (8): 428–31. PMID 9830392.

[101] McElhatton PR (1994). "The effects of benzodiazepine use during pregnancy and lactation". *Reprod. Toxicol.* **8** (6): 461–75. doi:10.1016/0890-6238(94)90029-9. PMID 7881198.

[102] Dolovich LR, Addis A, Vaillancourt JM, Power JD, Koren G, Einarson TR (September 1998). "Benzodiazepine use in pregnancy and major malformations or oral cleft: meta-analysis of cohort and case-control studies". *BMJ* **317** (7162): 839–43. doi:10.1136/bmj.317.7162.839. PMC 31092. PMID 9748174.

[103] Klein-Schwartz W, Oderda GM (January 1991). "Poisoning in the elderly. Epidemiological, clinical and management considerations". *Drugs Aging* **1** (1): 67–89. doi:10.2165/00002512-199101010-00008. PMID 1794007.

[104] Starr JM, Whalley LJ (November 1994). "Drug-induced dementia. Incidence, management and prevention". *Drug Saf* **11** (5): 310–7. doi:10.2165/00002018-199411050-00003. PMID 7873091.

[105] Inada K, Ishigooka J (January 2004). "[Dementia induced by antianxiety drugs]". *Nippon Rinsho* (in Japanese). 62 Suppl: 461–5. PMID 15011406.

[106] Lechin F, van der Dijs B, Benaim M (1996). "Benzodiazepines: tolerability in elderly patients". *Psychother Psychosom* **65** (4): 171–82. doi:10.1159/000289072. PMID 8843497.

[107] Wolkove, N.; Elkholy, O.; Baltzan, M.; Palayew, M. (May 2007). "Sleep and aging: 2. Management of sleep disorders in older people". *CMAJ* **176** (10): 1449–54. doi:10.1503/cmaj.070335. PMC 1863539. PMID 17485699.

[108] Tsunoda, K.; Uchida, H.; Suzuki, T.; Watanabe, K.; Yamashima, T.; Kashima, H. (Jan 2010). "Effects of discontinuing benzodiazepine-derivative hypnotics on postural sway and cognitive functions in the elderly". *Int J Geriatr Psychiatry* **25** (12): 1259–65. doi:10.1002/gps.2465. PMID 20054834.

[109] Hulse GK, Lautenschlager NT, Tait RJ, Almeida OP (2005). "Dementia associated with alcohol and other drug use". *Int Psychogeriatr* **17** (Suppl 1): S109–27. doi:10.1017/S1041610205001985. PMID 16240487.

[110] Wu CS, Wang SC, Chang IS, Lin KM (July 2009). "The Association Between Dementia and Long-Term Use of Benzodiazepine in the Elderly: Nested Case-Control Study Using Claims Data". *Am J Geriatr Psychiatry* **17** (7): 614–20. doi:10.1097/JGP.0b013e3181a65210. PMID 19546656.

Chapter 3

Text and image sources, contributors, and licenses

3.1 Text

- **Alprazolam** *Source:* https://en.wikipedia.org/wiki/Alprazolam?oldid=689136686 *Contributors:* Alex.tan, MadSurgeon, William Avery, Ewen, Someone else, Edward, Kadooshka, DopefishJustin, Collabi, Ixfd64, Delirium, Iluvcapra, Goatasaur, Ahoerstemeier, Angela, LittleDan, Ugen64, Jukeboksi, Thue, Owen, Nufy8, Fredrik, Moncrief, Yelyos, Hadal, JesseW, ElBenevolente, Cyrius, Jeremiah, Alexwcovington, DocWatson42, Ferkelparade, Marcika, Peruvianllama, Everyking, Jfdwolff, Guanaco, St3vo, Eequor, Matthäus Wander, Golbez, Gyrofrog, Andycjp, CryptoDerk, Slowking Man, Antandrus, Lockeownzj00, Jossi, Russell E, DragonflySixtyseven, RayBirks, Mysidia, Rlcantwell, Jollino, Joyous!, Daevatgl, Welte, Trevor MacInnis, PRiis, MattKingston, Diagonalfish, Blanchette, Rich Farmbrough, Cacycle, ArnoldReinhold, JPX7, Paul August, Bender235, Mykhal, Kbh3rd, Jarsyl, Mavromatis, El C, Kwamikagami, Pilatus, Causa sui, Bobo192, Reene, Longhair, Func, BrokenSegue, Arcadian, ToastieIL, Sasquatch, Llywelyn, Pacula, Googie man, Wayfarer, Agjchs, Alansohn, Arthena, Rd232, Avkrules, Jeltz, Dachannien, Aza-Toth, Calton, Axl, Malo, Velella, SidP, L33th4x0rguy, Helixblue, Cburnett, Tony Sidaway, Zumbojo, Cheyinka, Bsadowski1, Mattbrundage, Redvers, Agquarx, Djsasso, Dan100, Ceyockey, Galaxiaad, Tariqabjotu, Kelly Martin, Alvis, Woohookitty, GVOLTT, The Brain, JeremyA, MONGO, Kelisi, Tomlillis, Graham87, Magister Mathematicae, Kalmia, BD2412, FreplySpang, BorisTM, RxS, DePiep, Reisio, Canderson7, Rjwilmsi, Brianopp, PinchasC, Brighterorange, Krash, Bartelmask, AySz88, Sango123, Platypus222, Titoxd, Ian Pitchford, Margosbot~enwiki, Nihiltres, AI, Skillz187, Gurch, RobyWayne, Stevenfruitsmaak, Wgfcrafty, Bmicomp, Physchim62, WiccaIrish, RJSampson, Bgwhite, Digitalme, NSR, Gwernol, YurikBot, Xcali, NuMessiah, Sceptre, Midgley, RussBot, Petiatil, Jtkiefer, Anonymous editor, Tunafizzle, Inaniae, Pepijn Koster, C777, Gaius Cornelius, Tavilis, Remember me, NawlinWiki, Obarskyr, NickBush24, Aaron Brenneman, Banes, Rmky87, Drguttorm, Marc44, Rhodekyll, Samir, Derek.cashman, Delos~enwiki, Elkman, Smaines, Zzuuzz, Where next Columbus?, Chase me ladies, I'm the Cavalry, Theda, SMcCandlish, Dspradau, Colin, Skullfission, GraemeL, JoanneB, Cffrost, Spliffy, Tsiaojian lee, Katieh5584, Kungfuadam, Lyrl, 1231232, Moravek, Samuel Blanning, Saikiri, Mfigroid, Krótki, Crystallina, Frankie, SmackBot, GBarnett, Twerges, David Kernow, Pgk, Kilo-Lima, Jrockley, Arny, Edgar181, Shai-kun, Brianski, Ohnoitsjamie, Wlmg, Rearden Metal, TimBentley, Myxsoma, RDBrown, Hurricane Andrew, Ben.c.roberts, Rmt2m, Fuzzform, Deli nk, Dual Freq, Yanksox, Socraticus, Veggies, Zsinj, Can't sleep, clown will eat me, DHeyward, TheGerm, Skidude9950, TheKMan, Liberaljoe, Rrburke, Fantumz, BUF4Life, Naeboo, CWesling, ConMan, Cybercobra, Whaleto, Jwy, Nakon, TedE, Weregerbil, Drphilharmonic, DMacks, Evlekis, Wilt, Ohconfucius, Bige1977, Spiritia, Nathanael Bar-Aur L., Rory096, AThing, Attys, Microchip08, ER MD, Shadowlynk, Goodnightmush, Scetoaux, IronGargoyle, LebanonChild, Senseiwa, Slakr, Stwalkerster, Beetstra, Aeluwas, Mets501, Roregan, Geologyguy, NJA, KirrVlad, Dl2000, Beefyt, Hu12, Iridescent, Dockingman, JoeBot, Digitalsurgeon, Travis Myers, Dp462090, Marysunshine, Linkspamremover, Tawkerbot2, Ccroberts, Fvasconcellos, CmdrObot, Denverman, RedRollerskate, Harej bot, Ganfon, Seven of Nine, RobertLovesPi, JavaDog, Chq, TJDay, JediCarlos, Jac16888, Ntsimp, Chhajjusandeep, Bpekarev, MC10, Chasingsol, Retired user 0002, Christian75, RXPhd, Jerry Story, Javsav, PianoSpleen, Omicronpersei8, Mtijn, Jay.mccloud, Brock.enns, Casliber, Refault, Thegoodson, Thijs!bot, Qwyrxian, NoNamed, N5iln, Mojo Hand, Necrowarrio0, Headbomb, Marek69, Lark046, James086, Brichcja, JustAGal, Philippe, Mdriver1981, 0chiehchen, Mentifisto, AntiVandalBot, RobotG, Mr Bungle, Auoemski, Gamecheater2009, Wcbradley, Glockmeister, Stalik, Jcrock, Aspensti, JohnBigmen, Dallas84, John Cho, Deflective, Killfoot, MER-C, BranER, Bradleybox, VeronicaPR, MSBOT, Jwurm99, Typochimp, Garion333, Magioladitis, VoABot II, Yandman, Dinosaur puppy, Nyttend, Asaa00, Hhaassll, Sub40Hz, Indon, Farwestern, Tins128, Romancer, Su-no-G, Debollweevil, Alleborgo, JaGa, Edward321, Drmarilyn, Tiv83us, Rydra Wong, Tybalt01, WLU, Ebbinghaus, Yobol, ChemNerd, Edge79mi, Smilingsuzy, Nikpapag, R'n'B, Pbroks13, Discpad, J.delanoy, Captain panda, TimBuck2, AstroHurricane001, Nbauman, Darkride, Public Menace, Eliz81, Dspencer91, Spiperon, Jerry, Jodythomas, Little Professor, Williamcrobinson, Beelliott, Gefees, Mikael Häggström, Floaterfluss, Belovedfreak, Srpnor, SJP, Andreich2005, Dehughes, Cometstyles, STBotD, Sandtiger, HazyM, Mike V, Jarry1250, Jus1haz2, Aagtbdfoua, Squids and Chips, Thismightbezach, Idarin, Omegacc, IceJew, VolkovBot, TreasuryTag, CWii, Jeff G., Scorwin, Meth-Man47, Quentonamos, WOSlinker, Philip Trueman, TXiKiBoT, Knowledgebycoop, Rasotis, Devonspencer91, ZZuluZ, Rei-bot, Arnon Chaffin, Nazgul02, Briandavies80, PKDASD, Bodybagger, Markatl84, Cremepuff222, Georgegra, Maxim, RiverStyx23, Ghamer01, Hgjgfhj, Dvmedis, Carpetman2007, Paul gene, Enviroboy, Anna512, 51fifty, Orionvc, Doc James, Nagy, Snoopycool, Wesgarner, IndulgentReader, R.komorowski, BotMultichill, RJaguar3, Flyer22 Reborn, Tiptoety, Topher385, Olpres, Harashji, Oxymoron83, Crisis, Mr22, Dr. Doof, Spartan-James, Staciabb, Hamiltondaniel, Dosovits, Mikeeeee102, NBINVDR1, Vacanzeromane, Denisarona, Luke dm5, Tom Reedy, Literaturegeek, Chem-awb, Djfjwv, Troy 07, ImageRemovalBot, Iverson1, Atif.t2, Sfan00 IMG, Kazlow101, ClueBot, TJ Terry, The Thing That Should Not Be, Sonnycalhoun, FaShilio, ZFontaine, MikeVitale, Bigbillinsalmon, Wesleyx357, Mild Bill Hiccup, Jhaochen, Amit21pharma, Trivialist, JasWalker, Alexbot, Pdrcleaner, Wikitron22, 3bananas, Levelhand~enwiki, LevelTubes, Aettraffer, Nardog, Ssupak, MelonBot, Wnt, Attaboy, Editortothemasses, DumZiBoT, Italianstallion US, Klonster, Ean5533, XLinkBot, Openandshutcase, Arrowsmith36, Zeliboba, Facts707, SilvonenBot, NellieBly, Addbot, JBsupreme, C6541, Cantaloupe2, Wore Out Attorney, DOI bot, Issuevery, Viero666, TreasureXNY, Cssiitcic, Xmikemtxx, LaaknorBot, Favonian, Jasper Deng, 5 albert square, Esasus, Tide rolls, Gail, Megaman en m, Mackdaddymax, Luckas-bot, Nephro, Yobot, Tohd8BohaithuGh1, Legobot II, CheMoBot, Jadewasherejadewashere, Molepatrol, Rose bartram, RotogenRay, IW.HG, Sgtangie95, Magog the Ogre, Mnation2, AnomieBOT, Metalhead94, Casforty, Götz, IRP, Bflst1, Piano non troppo, Flewis, Materialscientist, Mrmz88, Monnish, Citation bot, Apfan, Qwerspam, ArthurBot, Quebec99, LilHelpa, Xqbot, Mongaakshay, TracyMcClark, Mononomic, Zethraeus, JWBE, حسن علي البط, GrouchoBot, Xasodfuih, ProtectionTaggingBot, Letsgoridebikes, Benjamin Dominic, Editor182, Pinetop18, The Sceptical Chymist, Custoo, Zacmea, VI, HJ Mitchell, Seer of Avalon, Citation bot 2, HamburgerRadio, Citation bot 1, Nirmos, SpaceFlight89, C7183235099c, BogBot, Niktzi222, Lotje, Dinamik-bot, Theo10011, David Hedlund, Iamcorey, Tbhotch, Ruskj, Minimac, DARTH SIDIOUS 2, Ams168, Onel5969, RjwilmsiBot, Ripchip Bot, Salvio giuliano, DASHBot, Bloodleech, EmausBot, Gfoley4, Rbaselt, Tommy2010, Joshuamcr, Dcirovic, Realxsalo, AvicBot, Josve05a, Felbutss, Mocceb, GZ-Bot, H3llBot, Semfaker, Weweta, Maddisonjack, 3DRivers, Mcmatter, Aschwole, SteveTyler, Sahimrobot, L Kensington, Rassnik, Half pint 707, DemonicPartyHat, Xianhua, Louisajb, ClueBot NG, This lousy T-shirt, Piast93, Pashihiko, Chester Markel, Irun42000, Xavier4075, Zaiazepam, Weed4201609, Helpful Pixie Bot, BG19bot, Jacki Moon, The Mark of the Beast, MusikAnimal, Charleswallacecharleswallace, Davidiad, CVX59, Kriswmack, Mark Arsten, Vanischenu, MathewTownsend, Anbu121, Fylbecatulous, Fuse809, Mediran, 00AgentBond93, Gotgot44, Dexbot, Mogism, Privatewhit1, Pvo73, Archdiamond, Faizan, Qwertyasdf99, Gary Battle, Vaccinationist, Kc2749, Qwh, AuQuebec, Clr324, Garzfoth, Tsundoku, Merlin2001, Soranoch, Meteor sandwich yum, 757crl, Bloggz1, Batcountrypdx, Monkbot, Renamed user 51g7z61hz5af2azs6k6, Mikzsan, JoshG1977, Apgloria, Asthuynh, Amypinsker1313, Zqp, Xlautolpbilea, Buymedicationsonline, Amortias, Medgirl131, A8v, Aethyta, Phoenix1961, Kuzunchev33, Denispolo, Arnold ganapathi, نينا سميث, April0318, AAhmedi FCS and Anonymous: 1080

- **Benzodiazepine** Source: https://en.wikipedia.org/wiki/Benzodiazepine?oldid=689406805 Contributors: AxelBoldt, TwoOneTwo, Kpjas, Bryan Derksen, RoseParks, RTC, Ixfd64, TakuyaMurata, Skysmith, Kosebamse, Ahoerstemeier, Jimfbleak, Kingturtle, BigFatBuddha, Cyan, Rob Hooft, LordK, Arteitle, Cheran~enwiki, Blainster, Sunray, Wereon, Fuelbottle, Diberri, Nagelfar, DocWatson42, Karn, Ich, Everyking, Michael Devore, Jfdwolff, APatcher, DO'Neil, Mboverload, Eequor, Foobar, DryGrain, Bobblewik, Isidore, Decoy, Chowbok, Andycjp, Slowking Man, Quadell, Antandrus, Russell E, Oneiros, Sharavanabhava, Rlcantwell, Publunch, WOT, Corti, Mike Rosoft, Alexrexpvt, Rich Farmbrough, Cacycle, Rama, Pie4all88, Petersam, MisterSheik, Kwamikagami, Dennis Brown, Wisdom89, Arcadian, La goutte de pluie, Alphax, MPerel, Wayfarer, HasharBot~enwiki, Jumbuck, Disneyfreak96, Agjchs, Alfanje~enwiki, Mo0, Eric Kvaalen, Wouterstomp, Thoric, Axl, Seans Potato Business, Pion, Bart133, Knowledge Seeker, Danhash, Evil Monkey, Mikeo, SteinbDJ, Stemonitis, Aerowolf, Bignoter, Tabletop, Dolfrog, Sherpajohn, Graham87, Kalmia, BD2412, DiamonDie, Reisio, Pmj, Rjwilmsi, Ian Lancaster, Brighterorange, The wub, FlaBot, Nihiltres, Dogbertd, RexNL, Bennett88, RobyWayne, Nicolay, Salvadorjo~enwiki, Stevenfruitsmaak, Overand, Physchim62, The Rambling Man, YurikBot, Wavelength, Edward Wakelin, Zafiroblue05, Rada, Gaius Cornelius, Kimchi.sg, Rmky87, Drguttorm, Tony1, Rhodekyll, Bilz0r, Derek.cashman, Jff119, Colin, GraemeL, TomHawkey, Andrew73, Scolaire, SmackBot, Brammers, Steve carlson, Reedy, Ifnord, Arny, Edgar181, Yamaguchi??, Brianski, Hraefen, Amatulic, Chris the speller, Davekrasmussen, Fuzzform, Moshe Constantine Hassan Al-Silverburg, Uthbrian, Socraticus, Wyckyd Sceptre, Can't sleep, clown will eat me, Petlif, Metallurgist, Yortek98123, Snowmanradio, Potnuru, Adamantios, Huon, Fuhghettaboutit, Pwjb, Drphilharmonic, Acdx, SashatoBot, Chaldean, Lambiam, AThing, Chazchaz101, Alan daniel, Slowmover, Robertg9, Joelmills, TheDapperDan, Beetstra, Renwick, SandyGeorgia, Mets501, Norm mit, Iridescent, Wwallacee, Noodlez84, PaddyM, BrOnXbOmBr21, Filelakeshoe, ChrisCork, Fvasconcellos, JForget, Denaar, CmdrObot, Todd Johnston, Flea392, Nunquam Dormio, Leevanjackson, TVC 15, Outriggr (2006-2009), Johnordq, Seven of Nine, Meodipt, Johner, Ispy1981, Alexandrelucas, Timeshift9, Anthonyhcole, Myscrnnm, Javsav, Surly Dwarf, Picard777, Casliber, Mattisse, Thegoodson, Thijs!bot, Bllix, Loudsox, Mojo Hand, Anupam, Kevinvlah, Headbomb, Rosarinagazo, John254, Mmcknight4, LAParker, Nick Number, Klausness, ThomasPusch, Escarbot, Hmrox, Trlkly, AntiVandalBot, RobotG, Mr Bungle, Has4, Christinedoby, Mzyxptlk, Wcbradley, TimVickers, Quihn, KMeyer, John Cho, JAnDbot, Deflective, MER-C, Srinivasan@physiology.wisc.edu, VeronicaPR, Patricknewyork, Magioladitis, Hroðulf, MastCell, Yandman, GridEpsilon, Crazytonyi, Fermentor, Caesarjbsquitti, Catgut, WhatamIdoing, Theroadislong, Tins128, WLU, Benzobuddy, Paulruiz, Rickard Vogelberg, TheRealGoozy, MartinBot, ChemNerd, Tremello, WotherspoonSmith, PGRandom, Xand3r, Leyo, Lilac Soul, JBC3, Tmallard, Boghog, Terrek, Ginsengbomb, Spiperon, Olivier Jaquemet, Aks4896, Ncmvocalist, Crallinz, Mikael Häggström, Wedgeantilles, Spinach Dip, Belovedfreak, Rev. John, ULC, A.Arc, Babedacus, The Right Honourable, Eionm, Lrunge, Jbo4, Lwalt, TreasuryTag, Charlycrash, Sdsds, Fluoborate, TXiKiBoT, Mercurywoodrose, Technopat, Nscc666, Arnon Chaffin, Garrondo, OyeMiCanto33, ^demonBot2, Pgdridge, Shanata, Eubulides, Benzowithdrawal.com, Carpetman2007, Lova Falk, Eartzi, Burntsauce, Doc James, BenzoBuddies, Rock2e, HkQwerty, Bakerstmd, Alextimmons, SieBot, MunkyJuce69, Gerakibot, Proevolution48, Benzoss, Monadyne, JasonOnEarth, Flyer22 Reborn, Grignardmonster, Oxymoron83, Kumioko, Husamymd, Scottyoak2, Dabomb87, Wenceslas23, Snoopycool2, Literatureegeek, Caspiax, Velvetron, Tatterfly, Kazlow101, Delighted eyes, ClueBot, LAX, Artichoker, Sonnycalhoun, EoGuy, ImperfectlyInformed, Politicalchalk, Mild Bill Hiccup, Vsbf, Epsilon60198, Michał Sobkowski, Crazyswedishguy, Peter.C, Medos2, Iohannes Animosus, Hans Adler, M.O.X, Zelda911111, Zahnrad, PCHS-NJROTC, Katanada, MelonBot, MasterOfHisOwnDomain, Danjgregory, DumZiBoT, AlanM1, XLinkBot, Arrowsmith36, Vanished 45kd09la13, Dthomsen8, Mjpresson, Svadhisthana, Coffee joe, Addbot, Vanished user zdkjeirj3i46k67, JBsupreme, Helvildfrisk, C6541, DOI bot, Stilldoggy, Ronhjones, Nomad2u001, TreasureXNY, Crisis counselor, Diptanshu.D, Looie496, Cst17, Mehryarj, AnnaFrance, LemmeyBOT, LinkFA-Bot, Jarble, WarmRegards, Legobot, Sagearbor, Luckas-bot, Yobot, Legobot II, AnomieBOT, Captain Quirk, Jim1138, Redskies08, Bluerasberry, Materialscientist, Citation bot, LilHelpa, Xqbot, TracyMcClark, Harbinary, Doctor1961, Loren1979, Giventends01, Letsgoridebikes, Argos42, REACHist, Shadowjams, Editor182, WaysToEscape, Anonabyss, The Sceptical Chymist, Legobot III, Prari, FrescoBot, Maasje, Rover Didn't Roll Over, D'ohBot, Julcal, Citation bot 1, PigFlu Oink, Nirmos, Jonesey95, Trappist the monk, عقیل کاشف, JessieTech, David Hedlund, RjwilmsiBot, Ochofive, TSChymist, Ripchip Bot, Wintonian, Bloodleech, Whywhenwhohow, EmausBot, John of Reading, Jpoulsen, Klbrain, Sallyb66, Tommy2010, Wikipelli, Dcirovic, Josve05a, Guitchounts, GZ-Bot, H3llBot, Donner60, Peteb4, RasmiG, Peter Karlsen, Unkept, Tejas320, Rocketrod1960, ClueBot NG, Ericobnn, Frietjes, Braincricket, CaroleHenson, Boyajian, Widr, OKIsItJustMe, Helpful Pixie Bot, Joint Nursing students AUS, BG19bot, Yuasan, Jay8g, Hope1967, Exercisephys, Fuse809, BattyBot, Ossip Groth, Jimw338, ChrisGualtieri, 32cllou, Khazar2, Jpkelada, SpacedOut84, Dexbot, Chrisandbev, Kingofdastreets1234, Mr. Guye, Cerabot~enwiki, Catclock, Naturedr, San Jaime, Ozzie10aaaa, Epicgenius, Qwertyasdf99, Camyoung54, DavidLeighEllis, Clr324, SwampFox556, Brainiacal, OccultZone, Anrrusna, Meteor sandwich yum, Yacine Er, Gazib184, Pigpie45, Monkbot, Renamed user 51g7z61hz5af2azs6k6, Akram1988, DocJulian, SailorMoon91, The Crappy Scientist 2013, BernardF111, Jeanjeni, Medgirl131, Aethyta, Mrs. Kringle, Philipjansen89, Jtxxtj, Youniszainal, Corpuskrusty, Size-

3.1. TEXT

ofint, KasparBot, Bossman Steve, Mahhon and Anonymous: 458

- **Anxiolytic** *Source:* https://en.wikipedia.org/wiki/Anxiolytic?oldid=689310348 *Contributors:* TwoOneTwo, The Anome, Fubar Obfusco, TomCerul, Edward, Ixfd64, MarcusAurelius, Julesd, Tristanb, Zoicon5, Defenestration, Ich, Eequor, Queerwiki, Chowbok, Andycjp, DragonflySixtyseven, Lazypplunite, Canterbury Tail, Gordonjcp, Discospinster, Rich Farmbrough, ESkog, CanisRufus, Arcadian, NickSchweitzer, Pearle, PatrickFisher, Dachannien, Malo, SidP, Stephan Leeds, Wadems, Galaxiaad, Notcarlos, SCEhardt, Graham87, Rjwilmsi, WiccaIrish, Jayme, YurikBot, Chris Capoccia, Lavenderbunny, Anomie, BOT-Superzerocool, Octavio L~enwiki, Feyandstrange, TTile, SmackBot, David Kernow, ScottWeston, Unyoyega, Ifnord, Jfurr1981, Edgar181, Cazort, Brianski, Benjaminevans82, Ohnoitsjamie, Ppntori, Amatulic, Brinerustle, T00h00, Drphilharmonic, Ohconfucius, JorisvS, Aum 101, Poweron, Salvinian, Devourer09, CmdrObot, 137 0, Linberry, Supposed, LastBall, Mattisse, Epbr123, Roadkill1984, Who123, Headbomb, CharlotteWebb, Heroeswithmetaphors, Mmortal03, FrRob, JAnDbot, Bahar, KonradG, WhatamIdoing, Tins128, Retroneo, Coffeepusher, Nikpapag, R'n'B, Ian.thomson, Inquam, DarwinPeacock, STBotD, Nikkilefevers, Lasombra bg, Sdsds, TXiKiBoT, O.mangold, Rei-bot, Doc James, Meldor, Alexbrn, Hxhbot, Yerpo, Xe7al, Stfg, Literaturegeek, Upisaida, Martarius, Sfan00 IMG, The Thing That Should Not Be, ImperfectlyInformed, Kmanclover, Wolfbeast, Nagika, MelonBot, DumZiBoT, Tigereye440, Vanished 45kd09la13, Brybryward, Facts707, Addbot, DOI bot, Download, Setwisohi, Yobot, Ptbotgourou, Mnation2, AnomieBOT, Metalhead94, Citation bot, Akapl619, Xqbot, Harbinary, 9468conleyd, PsychCat, Recognizance, Adlerbot, Jonesey95, Cinderchild, David Hedlund, Mramz88, RjwilmsiBot, DASHBot, EmausBot, John of Reading, Perfect Introvert, Dcirovic, Jodw~enwiki, Evasivo, Hazard-SJ, AManWithNoPlan, Erianna, Cornell92, Brycehughes, Rocketrod1960, ClueBot NG, Hadel.tabayoyong, Helpful Pixie Bot, Yuasan, Saturn 56, Gomada, J991, Aglo123, Wikijee, Fuse809, ChrisGualtieri, Makecat-bot, ⌘⌘⌘⌘⌘⌘⌘, Themoreyouno, LiamJamesBen, MV360, Clr324, Garzfoth, Patel manish22002, Monkbot, Djoce1, Roshu Bangal, Medgirl131, Mitchell328, Geene69, Robertovilla and Anonymous: 151

- **Benzodiazepine overdose** *Source:* https://en.wikipedia.org/wiki/Benzodiazepine_overdose?oldid=669941985 *Contributors:* DocWatson42, Rich Farmbrough, Arcadian, Rjwilmsi, Nihiltres, Ahpook, SmackBot, Drphilharmonic, DMacks, Fvasconcellos, DangerousPanda, Outriggr (2006-2009), Casliber, Mr Bungle, VeronicaPR, T@nn, Scottalter, Yobol, Hatf6, Coder Dan, Doc James, Literaturegeek, Drmies, MatthewVanitas, Diptanshu.D, Yobot, AnomieBOT, Africantearoa, Citation bot, Letsgoridebikes, Sophus Bie, Citation bot 1, PigFlu Oink, Der Elbenkoenig, Trappist the monk, RjwilmsiBot, GoingBatty, Brosef995, Helpful Pixie Bot, Sebastian80, MrBill3, RedGKS, CrunchySkies, TheOneHonkingAntelope, Qwertyasdf99, DendroNaja, Anrnusna, Monkbot, Julietdeltalima and Anonymous: 23

- **Benzodiazepine dependence** *Source:* https://en.wikipedia.org/wiki/Benzodiazepine_dependence?oldid=689231386 *Contributors:* William Avery, Rich Farmbrough, Bender235, Arcadian, RainbowOfLight, Guy M, Tabletop, Rjwilmsi, Ground Zero, Nihiltres, Tedder, Pigman, Rincewind42, Rsrikanth05, Fnorp, SmackBot, Yamaguchi⌘⌘, GoneAwayNowAndRetired, Chris the speller, Cybercobra, Drphilharmonic, Acdx, ArglebargleIV, JHunterJ, Smith609, Eastlaw, Cydebot, Chhajjusandeep, DumbBOT, Nsaum75, Headbomb, Nick Number, KrakatoaKatie, Christinedoby, BatteryIncluded, R'n'B, Boghog, Boskoman, Prhartcom, Coder Dan, Doc James, Mwalla, Literaturegeek, Dlrohrer2003, ClueBot, Arjayay, Cory Donnelly, MelonBot, Mjpresson, MystBot, ESO Fan, Addbot, Queenmomcat, Ronhjones, Diptanshu.D, SpBot, Luckasbot, Yobot, AnomieBOT, Go slowly, Citation bot, LilHelpa, Xqbot, A dullard, Letsgoridebikes, Aaron Kauppi, Citation bot 1, DrilBot, I dream of horses, Jonesey95, AHelpfulCommentator, Trappist the monk, Woodlot, RjwilmsiBot, Bloodleech, John of Reading, Dewritech, GoingBatty, Klbrain, Everything Else Is Taken, ZéroBot, AManWithNoPlan, Cornell92, Peter Karlsen, Guillaume0320, FiachraByrne, Widr, Helpful Pixie Bot, Joint Nursing students AUS, BG19bot, Yuasan, JohnChrysostom, BattyBot, Khazar2, GammaUpsilonRho, ⌘⌘⌘⌘⌘⌘⌘, Qwertyasdf99, Editor2286, Anrnusna, Ziva 84, Onlyevidence, Monkbot, Vatadoshu, Time3444 and Anonymous: 45

- **Benzodiazepine withdrawal syndrome** *Source:* https://en.wikipedia.org/wiki/Benzodiazepine_withdrawal_syndrome?oldid=687619529 *Contributors:* William Avery, Jtoomim, David spector, Skysmith, NuclearWinner, Jjshapiro, Chowbok, Etymancer, Neutrality, Rich Farmbrough, Bender235, Arcadian, RainbowOfLight, Guthrie, Ceyockey, Woohookitty, BD2412, Jclemens, Rjwilmsi, Cassowary, Nihiltres, Ewlyahoocom, Mathrick, Franko2nd, Marshalbyref, Pigman, Chris Capoccia, Skidoo, Wknight94, Deville, SmackBot, Brianski, Ohnoitsjamie, Chris the speller, RDBrown, Deli nk, CSWarren, Colonies Chris, Jmak, Acdx, Clicketyclack, Ohconfucius, ArglebargleIV, Eastlaw, VoxLuna, Erik Kennedy, ShelfSkewed, Seven of Nine, Cydebot, Chhajjusandeep, A876, Anthonyhcole, Alaibot, Curtvdh, Thegoodson, Headbomb, SGGH, Trlkly, SummerPhD, Aspensti, Struthious Bandersnatch, Lady Mondegreen, ChemNerd, R'n'B, Silverxxx, Captain Infinity, 1000Faces, Mikael Häggström, Belovedfreak, Trilobitealive, Mike V, Vinsfan368, Signalhead, Jmrowland, TXiKiBoT, Coder Dan, Guillaume2303, Seraphim, Ihowell67, Carpetman2007, Lova Falk, Doc James, Dawn Bard, Russcole, Techman224, Literaturegeek, Tatterfly, RobinHood70, Kazlow101, ClueBot, Dakinijones, Trivialist, Carusus, Callinus, MelonBot, George123me, XLinkBot, Tony8ha, Mjpresson, Svadhisthana, MystBot, Addbot, Willking1979, DOI bot, Julietacalabrese, Stilldoggy, TreasureXNY, Diptanshu.D, Esasus, Tassedethe, OlEnglish, Quisqualis5, Molepatrol, Rose bartram, AnomieBOT, Fangrah, Zawer, Citation bot, LilHelpa, Xqbot, Gigemag76, Letsgoridebikes, Ian Gottherd, Thehelpfulbot, FrescoBot, Wikinikistiki, Citation bot 1, Phearson, Trappist the monk, Lb.at.wiki, Taftster, RjwilmsiBot, John of Reading, GoingBatty, Klbrain, Crazyhorse77, Realxsalo, PBS-AWB, Xtzou, Cobaltcigs, Peter Karlsen, ClueBot NG, Delusion23, Layniek4172, FiachraByrne, Harris498, Faxigal, Bibcode Bot, Joint Nursing students AUS, BG19bot, Yuasan, MusikAnimal, Auqakuhreina, RichardMills65, StarryGrandma, Arcandam, Khazar2, Blessed Sky, Professor SWILUA, ⌘⌘⌘⌘⌘⌘⌘, Qwertyasdf99, Ruby Murray, ZXCV1234, Clr324, Thierry Le Provost, Wolololol, Jeremyregan, J.C.FMS1995, Onlyevidence, Monkbot, DigitalNoesis, Bdinker, QueenFan, Julietdeltalima, Vatadoshu, Penguinmlle, Truthforever 1234, Freemeat, Enough322, Dick tommygun, Factsfirst111 and Anonymous: 118

- **Benzodiazepine misuse** *Source:* https://en.wikipedia.org/wiki/Benzodiazepine_misuse?oldid=680995006 *Contributors:* DocWatson42, Robodoc.at, Daniel Brockman, Andycjp, Rich Farmbrough, Xezbeth, JoeSmack, Arcadian, Skrewler, Woohookitty, BD2412, Rjwilmsi, Nihiltres, Pigman, Gaius Cornelius, Daystrom, SmackBot, Gilliam, Chris the speller, Colonies Chris, Acdx, Ohconfucius, Kimholder, Eastlaw, Fvasconcellos, Cydebot, VeronicaPR, EagleFan, R'n'B, CommonsDelinker, Adavidb, Eionm, Cosmic Latte, Doc James, Moonriddengirl, Literaturegeek, QuintBy, Arjayay, Quetzapretzel, 7, Callinus, InternetMeme, Dthomsen8, C6541, BrianKnez, OlEnglish, AnomieBOT, Metalhead94, Citation bot, LilHelpa, 223fms, Bigtexpharmd, FrescoBot, Citation bot 1, AHelpfulCommentator, Orenburg1, Trappist the monk, RjwilmsiBot, Jb0nez123, GoingBatty, Realxsalo, H3llBot, Helpful Pixie Bot, Yuasan, Sebastian80, MrBill3, Ices2Csharp, BattyBot, Khazar2, Jacobjohnward, Khimaris, Dexbot, Mogism, FZenov, Qwertyasdf99, Vaccinationist, DendroNaja, Penitence, Clr324, Seppi333, YiFeiBot, Ziva 84, Monkbot, DocJulian and Anonymous: 37

- **Effects of long-term benzodiazepine use** *Source:* https://en.wikipedia.org/wiki/Effects_of_long-term_benzodiazepine_use?oldid=687463956 *Contributors:* Rich Farmbrough, Kay Dekker, Richard Arthur Norton (1958-), Woohookitty, Mandarax, BD2412, Rjwilmsi, Ground Zero, Nihiltres, Pigman, Raquel Baranow, Grafen, Rathfelder, Twerges, Kledsky, Chris the speller, Bazonka, Jwy, Drphilharmonic, Acdx, BrownHairedGirl, Eastlaw, Cydebot, Anthonyhcole, JustAGal, Nick Number, Zeitlupe, R'n'B, Nono64, 1000Faces, Davehi1, Doc

James, Juoj8~enwiki, Literaturegeek, Mild Bill Hiccup, Sun Creator, SchreiberBike, Freelion, Staticshakedown, WikHead, Addbot, Mr0t1633, Ocrasaroon, TreasureXNY, OlEnglish, Jarble, Luckas-bot, AnomieBOT, AtlMartinB, 90 Auto, Citation bot, DynamoDegsy, Quebec99, LilHelpa, Xqbot, Twirligig, Letsgoridebikes, Rudimae, Spidey104, Hoganben, Trappist the monk, RjwilmsiBot, John of Reading, Yiq, Super48paul, GoingBatty, KIbrain, ZéroBot, AManWithNoPlan, Aschwole, ClueBot NG, FiachraByrne, Helpful Pixie Bot, Bookie988, Exercisephys, IluvatarBot, Sheeren, BattyBot, Khazar2, AutomaticStrikeout, Monkbot, Jettybean, Pharmacyuk, Praxeolitic and Anonymous: 42

3.2 Images

- **File:Addictiondependence1.png** *Source:* https://upload.wikimedia.org/wikipedia/commons/b/b1/Addictiondependence1.png *License:* Public domain *Contributors:* drugabuse.gov *Original artist:* Unknown
- **File:Alprazolam_ball-and-stick_model.png** *Source:* https://upload.wikimedia.org/wikipedia/commons/b/b0/Alprazolam_ball-and-stick_model.png *License:* CC BY-SA 4.0 *Contributors:* PubChem *Original artist:* Vaccinationist
- **File:Alprazolam_structure.svg** *Source:* https://upload.wikimedia.org/wikipedia/commons/3/31/Alprazolam_structure.svg *License:* Public domain *Contributors:* https://pubchem.ncbi.nlm.nih.gov/compound/2118 *Original artist:* Vaccinationist
- **File:Alprazolam_synthesis.png** *Source:* https://upload.wikimedia.org/wikipedia/commons/b/b4/Alprazolam_synthesis.png *License:* CC BY-SA 4.0 *Contributors:* Own work *Original artist:* Nuklear
- **File:Alprazolam_synthesis.svg** *Source:* https://upload.wikimedia.org/wikipedia/commons/9/9a/Alprazolam_synthesis.svg *License:* CC BY-SA 3.0 *Contributors:* Vectorization of Alprazolam synthesis.png *Original artist:* Nuklear; derivative work by Master Uegly
- **File:Ambox_important.svg** *Source:* https://upload.wikimedia.org/wikipedia/commons/b/b4/Ambox_important.svg *License:* Public domain *Contributors:* Own work, based off of Image:Ambox scales.svg *Original artist:* Dsmurat (talk · contribs)
- **File:American_Lady_Against_The_Sky.jpg** *Source:* https://upload.wikimedia.org/wikipedia/commons/7/72/American_Lady_Against_The_Sky.jpg *License:* CC-BY-SA-3.0 *Contributors:* Transferred from en.wikipedia *Original artist:* Kenneth Dwain Harrelson
- **File:Ativan05mg.jpg** *Source:* https://upload.wikimedia.org/wikipedia/commons/9/96/Ativan05mg.jpg *License:* CC BY-SA 3.0 *Contributors:* Own work *Original artist:* Nsaum75
- **File:Benzodiazepine3.png** *Source:* https://upload.wikimedia.org/wikipedia/commons/2/21/Benzodiazepine3.png *License:* Public domain *Contributors:* Own work *Original artist:* Boghog2
- **File:Benzodiazepine_a.svg** *Source:* https://upload.wikimedia.org/wikipedia/commons/4/4b/Benzodiazepine_a.svg *License:* Public domain *Contributors:* Own work *Original artist:* Boghog2
- **File:Bzr_pm.png** *Source:* https://upload.wikimedia.org/wikipedia/commons/6/6f/Bzr_pm.png *License:* Public domain *Contributors:* Own work *Original artist:* Boghog2
- **File:Chlordiazepoxide.svg** *Source:* https://upload.wikimedia.org/wikipedia/commons/5/55/Chlordiazepoxide.svg *License:* Public domain *Contributors:* Own work *Original artist:* Harbin
- **File:Chlordiazepoxidetabletsgeneric.JPG** *Source:* https://upload.wikimedia.org/wikipedia/commons/8/86/Chlordiazepoxidetabletsgeneric.JPG *License:* GFDL *Contributors:* My local pharmacy allowed me to photograph generic non brand named pictures of chlordiazepoxide capsules. I took a picture of them with mobile telephone camera. *Original artist:* It is self created by myself with a camera
- **File:Commons-logo.svg** *Source:* https://upload.wikimedia.org/wikipedia/en/4/4a/Commons-logo.svg *License:* ? *Contributors:* ? *Original artist:* ?
- **File:Development_of_a_rational_scale_to_assess_the_harm_of_drugs_of_potential_misuse_(physical_harm_and_dependence,_NA_free_means).svg** *Source:* https://upload.wikimedia.org/wikipedia/commons/b/ba/Development_of_a_rational_scale_to_assess_the_harm_of_drugs_of_potential_misuse_%28physical_harm_and_dependence%2C_NA_free_means%29.svg *License:* Public domain *Contributors:* Based on Development of a rational scale to assess the harm of drugs of potential misuse. *Original artist:* w:de:Benutzer:Dosenfant
- **File:Diazepam2mgand5mgtablets.JPG** *Source:* https://upload.wikimedia.org/wikipedia/commons/b/b7/Diazepam2mgand5mgtablets.JPG *License:* GFDL *Contributors:* My local pharmacy allowed me to photograph generic non brand named pictures of diazepam tablets. I took a picture of them with mobile telephone camera. *Original artist:* It is self created by myself with a camera
- **File:Edit-clear.svg** *Source:* https://upload.wikimedia.org/wikipedia/en/f/f2/Edit-clear.svg *License:* Public domain *Contributors:* The *Tango! Desktop Project*. *Original artist:*

  The people from the Tango! project. And according to the meta-data in the file, specifically: "Andreas Nilsson, and Jakub Steiner (although minimally)."
- **File:Flumazenil.svg** *Source:* https://upload.wikimedia.org/wikipedia/commons/1/10/Flumazenil.svg *License:* CC BY-SA 3.0 *Contributors:* Self-made using BKChem and Inkscape *Original artist:* JaGa
- **File:Flumazenil1.JPG** *Source:* https://upload.wikimedia.org/wikipedia/commons/9/9d/Flumazenil1.JPG *License:* CC BY 3.0 *Contributors:* Own work *Original artist:* James Heilman, MD
- **File:Folder_Hexagonal_Icon.svg** *Source:* https://upload.wikimedia.org/wikipedia/en/4/48/Folder_Hexagonal_Icon.svg *License:* Cc-by-sa-3.0 *Contributors:* ? *Original artist:* ?
- **File:GABAA-receptor-protein-example.png** *Source:* https://upload.wikimedia.org/wikipedia/commons/4/45/GABAA-receptor-protein-example.png *License:* Public domain *Contributors:* Transferred from en.wikipedia to Commons by Sreejithk2000 using CommonsHelper. *Original artist:* Chemgirl131 at English Wikipedia

- **File:Midazolam.JPG** *Source:* https://upload.wikimedia.org/wikipedia/commons/7/7e/Midazolam.JPG *License:* CC BY 3.0 *Contributors:* Own work *Original artist:* James Heilman, MD
- **File:Normison.jpg** *Source:* https://upload.wikimedia.org/wikipedia/commons/3/3c/Normison.jpg *License:* Public domain *Contributors:* I (Editor182 (talk)) created this work entirely by myself.
Original artist: Editor182 (talk)
- **File:People_icon.svg** *Source:* https://upload.wikimedia.org/wikipedia/commons/3/37/People_icon.svg *License:* CC0 *Contributors:* OpenClipart *Original artist:* OpenClipart
- **File:Portal-puzzle.svg** *Source:* https://upload.wikimedia.org/wikipedia/en/f/fd/Portal-puzzle.svg *License:* Public domain *Contributors:* ? *Original artist:* ?
- **File:Question_book-new.svg** *Source:* https://upload.wikimedia.org/wikipedia/en/9/99/Question_book-new.svg *License:* Cc-by-sa-3.0 *Contributors:*
Created from scratch in Adobe Illustrator. Based on Image:Question book.png created by User:Equazcion *Original artist:*
Tkgd2007
- **File:Rod_of_Asclepius2.svg** *Source:* https://upload.wikimedia.org/wikipedia/commons/e/e3/Rod_of_Asclepius2.svg *License:* CC BY-SA 3.0 *Contributors:* This file was derived from: Rod of asclepius.png
Original artist:
- Original: CatherinMunro
- **File:Side_effects_of_alprazolam.svg** *Source:* https://upload.wikimedia.org/wikipedia/commons/5/5e/Side_effects_of_alprazolam.svg *License:* Public domain *Contributors:* All used images are in public domain. *Original artist:* Mikael Häggström
- **File:Speaker_Icon.svg** *Source:* https://upload.wikimedia.org/wikipedia/commons/2/21/Speaker_Icon.svg *License:* Public domain *Contributors:* ? *Original artist:* ?
- **File:Unbalanced_scales.svg** *Source:* https://upload.wikimedia.org/wikipedia/commons/f/fe/Unbalanced_scales.svg *License:* Public domain *Contributors:* ? *Original artist:* ?
- **File:Xanax_0.25,_0.5_&_1_mg.jpg** *Source:* https://upload.wikimedia.org/wikipedia/commons/b/bd/Xanax_0.25%2C_0.5_%26_1_mg.jpg *License:* Public domain *Contributors:*
- Xanax 0.25 mg tablets *Original artist:* United States Department of Justice
- **File:Xanax_2_mg.jpg** *Source:* https://upload.wikimedia.org/wikipedia/commons/1/12/Xanax_2_mg.jpg *License:* Public domain *Contributors:* I (Editor182 (talk)) created this work entirely by myself.
Original artist: Editor182 (talk)
- **File:Yes_check.svg** *Source:* https://upload.wikimedia.org/wikipedia/en/f/fb/Yes_check.svg *License:* PD *Contributors:* ? *Original artist:* ?

3.3 Content license

- Creative Commons Attribution-Share Alike 3.0

Printed in France by Amazon
Brétigny-sur-Orge, FR

13252717R00058